UNDERSTANDING
STROKE

For patients, carers and
health professionals

by
ROSEMARY SASSOON
with contributions by
specialists in the field

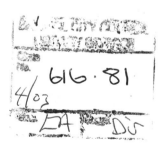
PARDOE BLACKER PUBLISHING

© 2002 Rosemary Sassoon

British Library Cataloguing in Publication Data:
A catalogue record for this book is available
from the British Library.

ISBN 1-897739-16-8

Published in the UK in 2002 by
Pardoe Blacker Publishing Limited
20 Copthorne Road
Felbridge, East Grinstead
Sussex RH19 2NS

1 3 5 7 9 8 6 4 2

Set in Joanna
Designed and produced by
Pardoe Blacker Publishing Limited

Printed in the United Kingdom
by Henry Ling Limited
at the Dorset Press, Dorchester DT1 1HD

Contents

Introduction   *page* 7
Acknowledgements   10

Part 1

FROM THE PATIENT'S PERSPECTIVE

Chapter 1: Before   13
Chapter 2: Observations as a patient in hospital   20
Chapter 3: At home   30
Chapter 4: Progress and suggestions   39

Part 2

DIFFERENT PERSPECTIVES

Chapter 5: The part played by the contributors   57

Chapter 6: Physiotherapy: the importance of a physical
management plan – JANE CAST, *Community physiotherapist*   65

Chapter 7: Functional Electrical Stimulation – the
Odstock Dropped Foot Stimulator – PAUL TAYLOR AND
JANE BURRIDGE, *Department of Medical Physics and Biomedical
Engineering, Salisbury District Hospital*   72

Chapter 8: The Bobath Concept – MARGARET J MAYSTON,
Director of the Bobath Centre, London   79

Chapter 9: When words don't work – what to expect
from speech and language therapy – DEBORAH HARDING,
West Kent Neuro-Rehabilitation Unit   84

Chapter 10: Cognitive problems following stroke –
KIT MALIA AND ANNE BRANNAGAN, *Defence Services Medical
Rehabilitation Centre, Headley Court*   97

Chapter 11: Different doctors – a personal view –
PROFESSOR D L MCLELLAN, Emeritus Professor of Rehabilitation,
University of Southampton and Past President, British Society of
Rehabilitation Medicine 105

Part 3
STROKE AND DIFFERENT AGE GROUPS: CHILDREN,
YOUNG ADULTS AND THE ELDERLY

Chapter 12: Different age groups 111

Chapter 13: Strokes in childhood – DR FENELLA KIRKHAM,
Paediatric Neurologist, Institute of Child Health 120

Chapter 14: The specific problems of younger stroke
survivors – DONAL O'KELLY, Founder of Different Strokes 127

Chapter 15: Some issues in stroke management for
the elderly – PROFESSOR KJERSTIN ERICSSON,
The Karolinska Institute, Department of Geriatric Medicine,
Huddinge Hospital, Stockholm 134

Part 4
RESEARCH

Chapter 16: An introduction to research 155

Chapter 17: Response-guided learning: research in
cognitive rehabilitation – BONNIE B CONNOR, DELROY
A HARVEY, R MARTYN BRACEWELL, GLYN W HUMPHREYS
AND ALAN M WING, Behavioural Brain Sciences Centre,
Birmingham University 158

Some final thoughts 179

Appendix. Information on the internet 180

Index 183

Introduction

RESEARCHING FOR THIS BOOK has made me realise how little I knew when I suffered my stroke and how much I would have liked to have such information myself when it was most necessary. In many cases, and in the first instance, it will be partners, parents or carers who might need to absorb and pass on the information included here, and the philosophy of hope and self-help that is propounded in the first part. But this book has a dual purpose, which will become clear as the reader progresses.

Patients need to understand their own condition and the role of the different health professionals they will encounter during their rehabiltation, and those nurses, therapists and even doctors need to understand more about the feelings and effects of the condition on their patients. This book is meant to be as relevant to them as to those they are treating. A successful outcome depends as much on a victory over the mind as over the body. I hope this will help to change some of the entrenched attitudes on the subject that hold back both patients' and professionals' expectations.

Many books about stroke suffer because the writers have not experienced a stroke themselves. They may be factually correct and useful but lack the insight that could bring them to life. Then there are those that are solely a personal report, enthralling and sometimes uplifting to read, but as strokes are so different in the way that they affect individuals, these may not be entirely relevant to patient, carer or health professional. It is hard to judge what is relevant to a reader in such a diverse subject. Patients' intelligence should not be underestimated. They and their carers deserve the highest level of information. Health professionals also would profit from as wide a perspective as possible on their patients' needs.

This book has evolved over a period of four years. It was two years after my stroke before I felt I had a balanced enough perspective of what had happened to record my observations. Over the next two years colleagues with whom I have worked in the past, alongside those who I have met during my recovery, have contributed their sections. As a result the contents of the book are divided between a personal report and some valuable professional perspectives. Although the range is wide, the concerns of every aspect of patient care cannot be fully discussed. It should, however, awaken readers to the many possibilities (and some of the problems) concerned with rehabilitation.

Nothing I have heard in the last couple of years from other patients, their carers, and parents of young children, or read during my recovery, has changed my view. Care and provision of information are regrettably patchy and often unsatisfactory. In the latest report from the Stroke Association, *Speaking Out About Stroke Services* (June 2001) one of the surveys indicated the particular need to meet the requirements of patients with psychological and psychiatric problems as a result of stroke. In that report one patient was reported as saying: 'Hospital staff should be made more aware of the variety of problems resulting from stroke. Sadly most disregard the feelings of patients and some even make fun of the situation'.

What happens in a crowded, understaffed geriatric ward is very different from the ideal put forward by the trainers of today's therapists. My feedback from patients all around the country has been about the lack of facilities and understanding of individual needs. Nothing that I have reported has been exaggerated, though I have concentrated on the National Health Service and not investigated private health care where undoubtably excellent care is obtainable in some places for those who can afford it.

You only need to read the informative publications from Different Strokes to understand that the plight of young stroke sufferers is even less addressed than that of the elderly. The situation of child stroke patients is no better understood. From those I come into contact with through my work in education, where their medical needs may, with luck, be adequately dealt with, their educational and psychological needs are seldom comprehended, much less met.

Much thought and planning is taking place at present into provision for the care of stroke patients. It still may take many years before enough young therapists and specialist nurses are trained – and more consultants and specialist doctors. With them will come the new attitudes towards their patients – because it is attitudes that need changing. That is just as important as more resources.

Acknowledgements

MY THANKS must first go to all the contributors: to friends I have worked with in the past, to those who contributed so much to my recovery and those I have met since – or have not yet had the pleasure of meeting. (The part they all played is explained in the book). They are all busy professionals who have written their chapters in the cause of disseminating knowledge to stroke survivors and their carers and sharing it with other health professionals. I owe a lot to many people in the various organisations, especially the Stroke Association, who patiently answered my queries and provided me with vital information. I think that I can safely say that there will be many readers who will also owe thanks to them.

I would like to thank Elwyn Blacker as well as his wife Jeanne Blacker. As both editor and publisher Elwyn encouraged me to complete this somewhat unconventional multi-level book – when others doubted if it could work. I must also thank Madaleine Combie who not only compiled the detailed index but also pointed out many inconsistencies in the text.

I would like to dedicate this book to my husband John, without whose loving care I would not have been able to make such a good recovery.

Part 1

FROM THE PATIENT'S PERSPECTIVE

CHAPTER 1

Before

FEW PEOPLE are lucky enough to have had any specialised knowledge to prepare them for the experience of
a sudden stroke. I was fortunate. Some years ago I
took part in a project at the suggestion of Alan Wing who
was then at the Medical Research Council Applied Psychology
Unit, Cambridge. He is now Professor of Human Movement
at Birmingham University (see page 178). It concerned
those who had lost the use of their natural writing hand –
the educational and medical aspects of handwriting being
my special interest at that time. It was intended to concentrate on the problems of directionality involved in having to
use the non-preferred hand. Stroke patients came into that
category as well as others suffering neurological impairment. The work was never published, but it served me very
well in the end as it brought me into contact for the first
time with those recovering from a stroke and those who
cared for them. This project seemed a logical extension of
my work with complex handwriting problems, but soon
showed that there were some unexpected benefits from using
handwriting to help in the retraining of a non-functional
hand. A presentation of this work at an Eastern Motor
Group meeting led to other contacts, and more patients. The
impressions I formed then were to affect my attitude to my
own recovery some fifteen years later.

Learning from patients

My small local hospital ran a stroke club about that time. It
seemed a good starting place for research. The speech therapist

who ran it ensured that her frail and elderly patients (mainly men) enjoyed their intensive speech therapy. There was a cheerful and positive atmosphere in the dark and dreary hut where the activities took place. It felt more like a social club than a hospital. However, in those days there were no occupational therapists working locally. I had a special interest in observing how patients were being retrained to write, but found that this was left to volunteer helpers – ladylike, caring but totally unskilled. Patients were encouraged to learn to write with their non-preferred, undamaged hand. Nothing was being done to help retrain their natural writing hand. They were being taught to use capital letters in the misguided assumption that they would find it easier. In fact, the constant repositioning of the pen required in the writing of capital letters is usually much more difficult for anyone getting used to their non- preferred hand. This also applies to anyone with a tremor, from whatever cause. It should be recommended only when the writer previously wrote solely in capital letters.

Case 1 taught me how some patients found their own solutions, even in the face of inappropriate advice. This also made me consider that it might actually be counter-productive to encourage the use of the non-preferred hand except when absolutely essential. The gradual return to the use of the right hand, in a way that was visible and could be monitored, would signal progress towards normality and might have an even deeper meaning to a patient.

An elderly man, who had suffered a stroke some two years before, was proudly presented as the group's most successful patient. He was indeed managing to write a passable script with his left hand. When asked if he had ever tried to write with his right hand the answer was: 'Of course I can write perfectly well now with my right hand but I haven't told the kind ladies here because they seem so pleased that they have taught me to use my left hand'. There seemed no understanding of the value of retraining his right (preferred) hand.

Dear Sir,
I am writing I am curling
Dear Sir
I am writing to you concerning

The patient's left-handed (*above*) and right-handed writing (*below*).

That man recounted something that many patients have mentioned since, that he did not feel that his left-handed writing was really a true representation of himself, and he only felt comfortable once he could return to his old writing, however shaky it was at first.

Case 2 gave me an opportunity to investigate how to use handwriting to be a visible and welcome sign of progress for patients themselves. The idea of using handwriting as an aid to diagnosis is far from original. This patient showed that the written trace could be a useful measure for health professionals to monitor returning motor function, and other aspects of a patient's condition. It showed unexpected additional benefits in countering depression and helped me to formulate my ideas about the effects of motivation on a patient's attitude to recovery.

It was the usual practice then to delay therapy for several weeks, so it was not easy to gain access to patients to assess the effect of early intervention. However, in a nearby nursing home, was a woman in her mid-forties who had just suffered her second stroke. A teacher, she despaired of ever returning to her profession. To show her that she would be able to write again seemed a first step towards regaining her confidence. There were no facilities at the hospital, so we borrowed a piece of hardboard and rested it at an angle against the bed as she sat by it. The patient was encouraged to make any mark she could with a felt pen, supporting her (considerably) damaged right hand with her left, in any way that was comfortable.

The illustration on the frontispiece shows how it is quite easy to make any stroke (in the graphic sense of the word) into the resemblance of some letter or other. In two or three sessions, over a period of about three weeks, this lady progressed to a passable signature – one of the most important things for any disabled person to acquire. It is the way you present yourself to the world. Without a signature, even with the advent of computers, you are forever dependent on someone else to deal with your business affairs if you are unable to fill in a form, or sign a cheque.

The therapists and nurses involved in this patient's care expressed astonishment at her progress. 'She could suddenly begin to use a knife and fork', said one. 'She even managed to open a window', said another the next week. It transpired that the only exercises that she would have been offered to improve hand function would have been to have two boxes and told to practise transferring buttons from one to another. This was hardly inspiring or motivating to an intelligent and distressed patient. Practising and watching the gradual improvement of your own script is quite another matter. The woman, with little else to do, was constantly striving to improve her signature, and in doing so made great strides in improving her hand function. What this did for her self-confidence and relief from depression was evident to us all.

Case 3 has considerable implications for those who despair because they have lost the ability to communicate, and for those who care for them. The point to make here is that because the power of speech is temporarily (or even permanently) impaired there is no reason to assume that the ability to write has been affected. It is always worth trying to see if the patient is still able to communicate through writing.

It was some years later, in Singapore, when a physiotherapist invited me to join her on her rounds. She wanted me to see a distinguished Chinese patient who did not seem to be making the progress that she had expected. She described how he had been an eminent public figure and had always dreaded becoming disabled and unable to communicate. In the position he now found himself, his worst fears had been realised. He lay motionless on the bed, not even trying to co-operate with the physiotherapist. I asked his nurse if he had been offered any kind of indicator board to help him to have some small degree of control, perhaps choice over his food or drink. The reply was that the hospital could not afford such luxuries, and I had to point out tactfully that all I meant was a piece of paper with some simple drawings on it.

I found myself asking if anyone had ever tried to find out whether the patient could write with his functional hand. This provoked an uproar, and some most unfortunate remarks by the nurse about the patient's mental state that, in her considered opinion, would preclude any such activity. One look at the patient's eyes made us realise that we had made a breakthrough. A piece of paper and a pencil were grudgingly found and the patient produced a perfect sequence of Chinese characters with his left hand. I never found out what he had written because none of us could read Chinese, but I heard later that, though confined to a wheelchair, the patient otherwise made a full recovery.

Case 4 illustrated the consequences of what can occur when appropriate treatment is not available. Strokes are not confined to the elderly, far from it. One young stroke patient, a boy of about nine years old, was brought to me by his teacher who was worried that he had problems trying to write with his left hand. It appeared that he had had very successful therapy for his right leg at a London teaching hospital, and no longer showed any signs of a limp. He was supposed to have had therapy for his arm after he returned home. For whatever reason, this had not taken place. He held his right arm behind him. He said it was his enemy, and that the children at school called him the one-armed bandit.

It seemed to me that there was no reason why he should not be able to retrain his right hand, and get it functional. I was only going to see him once so there was little time to find out. I sat him at the kitchen table and put a packet of chocolate biscuits in front of him and told him that he could take the first one with his left hand but then he must use his right one if he wanted any more. It was fascinating to watch him. His hand seemed to go through all the stages of development, but gradually he controlled the contortions, and by the end of the packet was quite efficient. It was then a short step to show him that he was perfectly capable of holding a pencil in his right hand, and with practise, he should be able to begin to write. But it was not to be. Another school year brought a change of teacher; it was later reported that, without further help or encouragement, frustration and behavioural problems set in.

Conclusions

These, and other patients helped me to formulate my ideas. Even though my area of research was specialised and somewhat limited, it seemed to me that all patients reacted positively to active motivation, especially to something with visual feedback. Encouragement roused them from their apathy and they all responded to being treated as intelligent people. It appeared that this had not always been the case. Their particular talents, their home environment and their future expectations all had to be considered. Then with practical, realistic encouragement, and the respect that everyone deserves, whatever therapy they received would be more effective. I saw evidence in some of the cases that came my way of the waste of human potential and the disastrous consequences of inadequate therapy, and depressing, ill-informed care. I was not particularly well informed about what might have been happening in major teaching hospitals and other centres of excellence, but my recent personal experiences and observations have not led me to change my mind.

My interest then shifted, to dystonia patients, investigating the problems of writer's cramp patients at several London hospitals over a period of five years. I had to acquire a little basic neurology, and during that time attended a few seminars and presentations – and occasionally gave them – but that was all the knowledge I brought with me to inform me when, somewhat ironically, I suffered a stroke one day after my sixty-seventh birthday.

CHAPTER 2

Observations as a patient in hospital

THE STROKE ASSOCIATION carried out an exhaustive survey in 1999 entitled: *Stroke Care – A Matter of Chance*. It reported that: 'More people suffering from strokes are now getting progressive and co-ordinated stroke care. But the most striking results show clearly the haphazard nature of access to this care. ... If patients do not have access to such care they are more likely to die, and if they survive are more likely to be disabled.' The *Daily Telegraph's* article *There is Life after Stroke* (13 April 1999) discussed this report, and again highlighted unacceptable regional variations, as well as delays and inadequacies that result in thousands of avoidable deaths and more disabilities for those who survive. It is not only articles like this, which went on to chronicle individual patients' experiences, but confirmation from many other sources that convinced me that my experiences and observations were not exceptional. I am not interested in implying criticism of hard-pressed National Health hospitals, but in analysing my impressions of how it felt to be a patient in such a way that it might be of interest or use to others.

The overriding need for all patients is to be informed and reassured – to understand what has happened to them and what is the likely outcome. It must be a terrifying experience to regain consciousness in a hospital, unable to move, unable to speak and with no understanding of what has occurred. From what I witnessed myself in hospital, the most unfortunate patients were those unable, even temporarily, to communicate. This is how one man explained what happened to him when he had a stroke in his late twenties: when he regained consciousness in a busy south London hospital he could neither move, speak or swallow. People talked about him, and over him in terms he could not comprehend. When, after about three days, he heard a doctor say that they could do no more for him, and to call an ambulance, he was quite convinced that he was going to be sent home to die. Needless to say he was being transferred to a rehabilitation unit and subsequently made a full recovery. Many years later he could still recall his anguish, and it upset him to talk about it. I was lucky, my stroke started slowly, I recognised what was happening even before I saw a doctor, and knew approximately what to expect – though, perhaps just as well, I had little idea of how long my recovery would take.

Motivation

The next imperative is for everyone involved in the care of patients to put as positive a slant as possible on everything, to provide encouragement and motivation. For most patients recovery is going to be a battle. If this is called a challenge then the emphasis is slightly altered. The sooner it is explained that the more you help yourself the better the outcome will be, the benefits of any therapy will be compounded. To be involved in your own recovery and be given partial responsibility for its success gives impetus, then every action becomes therapy. What you find difficult is what you can aim to improve. I do not want to make this chapter too much of a personal account, but some aspects may be of general interest.

Although I could not record my first impressions at the

time, they are still vivid. My right side was completely paralysed, other than a little movement in my fingers. Patients had, in the past, described to me the feeling when their bodies refused to obey the dictate of their brain, but to experience it is another matter. The terms 'neural plasticity' or 'the forging of new pathways' are often discussed and I knew my brain had to find new ways of producing a movement now the part that used to control that function was damaged. The normal channels did not work so I tried to 'think' my wrist to move. The way I would describe it is that at first there was no contact between me and my wrist. Amazingly, there was soon a quiver. I cannot remember how many days it was before I could raise my hand an inch from the bed, but the connection was made and only needed to be strengthened. I had a goal now, and the motivation to reinforce this quiver.

The term 'brain damage' has frightening connotations for the general public. Changing the term 'stroke' to 'brain attack', as is being suggested, may not make the matter much better. Patients need to understand their condition. That would be the first step towards motivating them to help themselves. Maybe it would be difficult for other than a neurologist to convey to stroke patients the wonderful capacity of our brain to reorganise, and not everyone would be able to comprehend. It is asking a lot, but a simple explanation might be a comfort and an encouragement to those for whom it seemed appropriate. Families also would benefit from a bit of hope in those early, distressing days.

Depression and tiredness

I recall an incongruous episode some time during my first few days in hospital. A pleasant young man in a white coat, perhaps a medical student, appeared at my bedside. He was carrying a clipboard and almost his first question was 'On a scale of 1 to 10 how depressed did I feel?' When I replied that I did not feel at all depressed this confused him as if there was no space to record an answer like that. Many, if not most, patients are depressed to some degree, and who can blame them. Apart from the shock of what they are experiencing at that moment, and their worries about the future, most people's perception of the results of a stroke are coloured by memories of an elderly, disabled, infirm relative. I witnessed some patients who were deeply troubled, and the over-worked nursing staff had little time to counsel them. Medication is obviously needed at the deeper levels of depression. However, I gained the impression that much could be done to alleviate some of the very genuine worries of these patients with a little thought. Someone could take the time to explain as simply and clearly as possible what was going to be done to help the patient and what they could do to help themselves. Even when the patient appears uncomprehending this is important. This is surely part of the training of all concerned nowadays, but in the rush and realities of a crowded ward it seems, from many people's experience, that this does not take place.

To complicate the issue, most stroke patients would agree that tiredness becomes a fact of life, in hospital and long after. Tiredness and lethargy can be confused with depression. You can fight it, moan about it or recognise the benefits sleep brings. You may be retraining every action that you once took for granted: your speech, of course, also the way you laugh, the way you yawn or sigh. Trying to dress is tiring, and any kind of therapy even more so. Visitors are tiring and often interrupt those times when you would be better resting, and letting your body assimilate what you have learned in therapy sessions.

Early intervention

When I had been doing my earlier work it had still been the policy to delay rehabilitation for a considerable time. I had formed a strong conviction that early intervention was desirable, if only to reassure patients. In the interest of describing good practice, this is what occurred that first morning, when, in a non-specialist ward, I asked to see a physiotherapist. The neuro-physiotherapist who appeared sized up the situation and drew some graphic diagrams in green felt pen. These she fixed above my bed to show every passing nurse how to straighten my limbs. The strategically placed pillows she recommended made a huge difference to my comfort.

The medical staff reacted positively to her pictorial instructions and I am convinced that the very early intervention was extremely valuable. It reminded me how the Singapore physiotherapist (see page 17) had stressed that one of her main jobs was straightening the limbs of her home-based patients and trying to train their relatives to do likewise. Until we have specialist stroke units in every district hospital, nursing staff need to know such common sense techniques.

I should add here that in my particular case I did not feel that it was a disadvantage being placed in the early stages in an orthopaedic ward, as in many cases it would be. First of all I knew what to ask for and found that excellent therapist. She also dealt with those first rather frightening days, trying to achieve as much as to enable me to stand up. But it was something else entirely that was the most help in coming to terms with what had happened. Everyone else was so cheerful. The atmosphere did not allow me to dwell too much on my troubles. Only too soon I was dispatched to a geriatric rehabilitation unit where the physiotherapy was of the same excellent standard – but the atmosphere depressing, even daunting.

The benefits of helping yourself

Patients need to understand that to help themselves in any way they can is the best way forward. From the beginning it would be beneficial even if it could be stressed how just a little stretching in bed to reach objects (instead of ringing for the nurse or doing without) would help.

At the acute stage patients may have to accept help with everything. However, even to start learning to dress yourself can be presented positively as useful therapy. It does not matter how long it takes to fasten a button, or make the reluctant fingers of a non-preferred hand support the inefficiency of the damaged one, if it is all related to a gradual recovery. Learning new strategies to dress will be tiring, and time consuming, but there is plenty of time. If it is all explained as therapeutic, then, as each task becomes a little easier, self-esteem and optimism will rise.

My attitude was not only influenced by thinking of the benefit to be gained by exerting myself a little more each day, but of a deep hate of being dependent. Dignity and privacy are hard to find on a busy ward. One of the selling points of private medical care is that it ensures privacy. That appeals to many people, but it denies you the camaraderie of the public ward, and sometimes the constant observation that you get in an acute NHS ward. When it comes to an emergency, and this includes a stroke, then the shock of a public ward is reinforced by this stereotypical concept of the desirability of a private room.

There are obvious tiresomenesses and indignities as a result of not being mobile. There are plenty of wheelchairs on any ward, but I noticed that patients were not encouraged to try to make use of them. When one day I was left in a wheelchair after a therapy session I tried it out around the ward. My efforts were greeted with surprise and by the remark: 'Our ladies never try to take themselves around and only a few of our men'. Apart from the immediate benefits, if patients are going to be wheelchair dependent as soon as they are released, it might be a good idea for them to have a bit of practice first.

Eating and drinking

Serious incidents of eating and drinking problems are recognised and dealt with – but I am not so sure about marginal ones – and they do affect the patient's confidence and wellbeing. Eating, with one side of the body out of action, is never going to be easy. In hospital there seemed to be little between total assistance with feeding and none at all. Those who could not communicate were again at a disadvantage. They had no choice in the matter of food or drink and, as so often, a simple indicator chart (tea/coffee, milk/sugar) might have helped.

I now know that swallowing is a common – and sometimes a serious – problem. The Stroke Association has a leaflet concerned with swallowing problems and I wish I had had access to it when I really needed to understand what was happening to me. I found it a couple of years later on a stand at an out-patient clinic. The leaflet starts by explaining that swallowing is a very complicated process involving many muscles. If any one of these is not working properly there may be a difficulty with eating and drinking, especially when combining solids and liquids. One of the first questions I was asked on admission was whether I could swallow. I obediently gulped, and not knowing any better, replied, yes. From that day onwards I was puzzled by the fact that I could usually swallow food, yet had difficulty with liquids. Being cheerful meant that it was assumed all was well, but long after returning home I had to contend with swallowing difficulties, and found it difficult to make myself drink enough. There were alarming occurrences of choking. Two years later I still have to be careful.

Dealing with spasms and cramps

There is not necessarily much pain after a stroke. There may be frightening experiences, like choking and there is another uncomfortable problem, another of the many issues that patients deserve to have explained to them. That is a mixture of involuntary movement, spasms and cramps due, I now realise, partly to the contraction of muscles, and not being able to turn over easily during sleep. These annoyances seemed at the time quite positive indicators of returning movement as they affected, most markedly, the parts of my body that were just becoming mobile. If rationalised that way they seemed quite welcome. Other patients confirm my own experience that these cramps and spasms may continue for many months or even longer. They would benefit from help with strategies to minimise the effect, such as avoiding too much stretching or any abrupt movements, straightening limbs very slowly and in small stages. Having a hot shower on waking is also a great help.

Record keeping for the patient's sake

A brief diary, whoever keeps it, might well help both patient and a partner or family to accept what is happening. I read with some envy of Robert McCrum's efforts in keeping a diary – and not only as an aid to writing his book My Year Off.* In the hospital where I treated most of my dystonia patients, their progress was recorded on video. This was intended for research and training purposes, but proved therapeutic for the patients. It enabled them to see how

* Picador 1998

much they had improved in a short period of time. When everything still seems grim, it may be difficult for stroke patients or their families to appreciate the progress that is being made, and it would give them encouragement. Maybe this technique is used in some rehabilitation units; if not it might be worth a try.

Preparing for release

A stroke patient has a lot of planning to do before undertaking any new action such as getting in and out of a chair, much less a car, and there is plenty to think about before returning home. How they will manage in the outside world is a major concern for many patients. For those who need it, the occupational therapists will pay a pre-release visit to their homes to advise on safety and other matters. There is usually an excellent service for lending out necessary equipment, wheelchairs, bath seat, etc. A care package can deal with such matters as delivering meals if necessary. In the interest of alleviating worry all this should be explained long before the patient is ready to leave.

Our hospital, in common with many, did not provide therapy sessions at the weekend. The staff were quite positive about letting those about to be released have a trial day at home (or even a night) beforehand. Contrary to many people's expectations, the hospital was in no hurry to discharge me. They made it quite clear by stressing that there was no time limit to my stay. My physiotherapist made it even clearer, warning me that I would be sacrificing my daily sessions for a very limited service 'outside'. Little did I know how limited it was to prove to be or I might have stayed another week or so – but it was Easter. To return after three days of freedom would not have been easy. It was the first of many issues that were to be balanced in the next few months – therapy and safety against motivation and functional improvement. In other words, would I progress more quickly at home with all the motivation to move and use my hand, free from the increasingly depressing atmosphere of what was becoming more of a general geriatric ward, with more of its share of dementia patients, than a rehabilitation unit? For those living alone or in unsuitable accommodation, the decision would have had to be different. I was deemed just about safe enough to transfer myself from chair to chair, and up the stairs, so with thanks but few regrets I was homeward bound the day before Good Friday. I had been in hospital for nearly two months.

CHAPTER 3

At home

AFTER THE INITIAL EUPHORIA of being back in your own home, there is a realisation that quite a lot of the habits of a lifetime will have to change. Those around you may also have to adjust their lifestyles. It will take a lot of planning and involve compromises on both sides – but most of all on yours. If you set out with the idea that you are going to improve and get back your mobility and independence as soon as possible, then it is not so bad to sit back a little and give up some of your former role in the home or elsewhere. Usually common sense will prevail as it becomes obvious that you are not yet able to do many things that you once took for granted. An optimistic outlook is essential to both patients and carers, but it is not easy to find the right balance in everything. Too much assistance may stifle initiative. It may risk sapping the patients' confidence in their ability to get better, and turn them into permanent invalids. Then, when the family loses confidence in their ability to cope, there is a risk of institutionalising elderly patients. After all, it is only by attempting and practising the very actions that you find difficult that you slowly improve.

Too little assistance and the whole system may fail in a different way. The patients might also lose all confidence in the future through constant failure. They might take too many risks and be in danger of falling, or become frustrated by the sudden limitations on their life. Once again it depends on so many factors. Within a marriage or steady relationship, for instance, the challenge of changing roles can result in anything from a disaster to a deeper understanding and satisfaction. The patient's partner needs consideration too, Having to take all the responsibility of home, family, and perhaps business as well as caring, is a heavy burden for anyone.

Compromise will be needed in many things – in shopping for instance, when you suddenly become dependent on someone else. It is amazing what you can manage without, with a bit of ingenuity. You will probably have to drop your standards temporarily, in many ways such as tidiness in the home, To ignore the rampaging weeds in the garden could be just as difficult for some people, as I found myself. It will be hard not to get frustrated, but in the circumstances there is not much else to do. Positive things may be happening all the time, as gradually a way of coping becomes clearer. A certain satisfaction comes when different strategies are found for dealing with some of the jobs in the home.

The contrast between in hospital and out

Most of these factors are obvious – the comfort of having your own bed once again, being able to use the phone, choose to a certain extent your own food, go to bed when you want and get up at a sensible time of day, turn on the radio or the TV – the list is endless. There is a down side though. This is common to many other conditions, not only stroke. You feel pretty vulnerable as you realise that everything is now up to you or your family. There may no longer be someone to call if anything goes wrong, if you fall or drop something vital and find it impossible to retrieve it. Your own clumsiness becomes more evident and breakages and the messes resulting from dropped meals and spilled drinks are almost inevitable. There may even be moments of real panic when you find yourself in a position that you cannot resolve.

There will be decisions large and small that need to be taken when you would rather sleep and forget about it all. Some people will understand how you feel, some may consider you unhelpful, even wilful, and some people will try and take over matters that you would rather they left alone. Whatever the situation you will be expected to be grateful. You have to learn to receive graciously and yet are unable to give – you have to learn fast, and it is not always easy. It helps you and all concerned if you are more courteous than usual. This may seem an odd thing to say, but I at least found it made me feel better.

Safety at home

The most important issue is safety. Assuming that you will already have the basic equipment to help you become as independent as possible, the planning can begin. The balance is always between going forward and keeping up your morale, and safety. A broken bone as the result of a fall can be devastating on top of neurological impairment.

Stairs can be a risky and tiring manoeuvre but it is often possible to plan so you do not have to undertake it more than once a day and, initially, not unattended. Later on the same sort of rule could be applied to going outside – not to venture forth unless someone is within hearing distance. It is far harder for anyone on their own to take the small risks that seem essential to functional progress. 'Mother would never have got out of her chair again unless one of us went in every day and encouraged her to walk up the garden,' said one acquaintance. What motivates a person to become mobile and independent must vary considerably. It may be to be able to visit grandchildren perhaps, a desire to go to church, to do your own cooking, to return to work, or sheer determination not to be defeated. As one person put it: 'My father hated what the stroke had done to him so much that he was determined to beat it'. Everyone needs a bit of encouragement if they are going to recover. Whatever the motivation it is going to mean hard work and patience – and perhaps imagination – on the part of all concerned.

Conserving energy

There is another compromise and that effects all aspects of daily life. Energy is likely to be limited so that a judgement has to be made as to whether it is worth expending it on any particular act. It is still there as stamina improves – there is always more that needs doing or you want to do than you will be able – or other people think you should do. That is true of all life in general, but in this situation it is just more obvious, and the effects more serious.

The effects of getting overtired could last several days. Movement, speech, memory and other factors can be temporarily affected by over-tiredness. There are likely to be all kinds of helpful suggestions from friends and family – therapy, alternative and conventional, that may be available only at a distance, beneficial or socially desirable activities, etc. However, to get to them would be far too tiring and time-consuming to justify their benefits. It is always necessary to listen to your body. Only the patient can judge whether any particular activity is worth getting exhausted for. One small warning. However energy consuming it may be it is not worth ignoring regular eye and dental checkups. They can easily be overlooked in the new situation with quite serious consequences.

Then there is the matter of different times of day. Mental and physical energy will vary according to the time of day. This can be affected by medication. Some people will progress during the day and become more stretched and flexible. They feel better in the evening and find it far easier and more effective to do exercises then. Things that they would not be able to do in the mornings because of being too stiff, work better then. Other people report the opposite. It is one more factor to notice and plan for so as to get the best out of each day. Extremes of heat or cold may affect a patient recovering from a stroke much more than in the past. Any small setback, such as a minor infection, can affect your progress. To be more accurate, it may cause you to regress and it is important to understand that what is happening is only temporary and not become discouraged.

Out-patient physiotherapy

The real difference between being an in-patient and an out-patient is therapy – no more comforting daily sessions, no more expert help and encouragement. I was warned on the ward that things would not be the same, but nothing prepared me for the limited and comparatively inexpert therapy I received from that day on. I realise now that that was probably just a local problem. Where we live, even if a patient could afford a private neuro-physiotherapist there was none nearby. I knew then that it was basically up to me whether I got better or not. The same situation seems to arise all over the country, according to dozens of other people I have talked to, and the consequences for those who do not know how to help themselves must be much more serious. Away from large cities and hospitals, few people seem to get adequate therapy once they leave hospital. It may vary from trust to trust, and the situation should improve, but I can only report my experiences in an affluent area of the south-east, from 1998 onward.

The whole treatment of stroke patients after they leave hospital can be seriously inadequate. The superficial explanation is that the NHS is underfunded; but there are several more issues involved. One is the relationship between doctor and therapist. Stroke patients are usually referred to the local physiotherapy service. Appeal to the GP is still possible, but then his or her remoteness and increasing lack of expertise make the need for intervention difficult to establish and its form difficult to prescribe. Once the stroke patient has left hospital and been referred for therapy, the GP has lost effective control. The selection and training (or retraining) of therapists does not always seem to have kept pace with the enlargement of their responsibilities. Large hospitals, with their concentration of acute patients and specialist equipment need, and are a magnet for, the most able therapists. As a result the quality of out-patient therapy, particularly neuro-physiotherapy, can vary widely. I suspect country areas suffer most.

Attitudes

Other people's attitudes cannot help but affect your confidence. The attitude of your general practitioner, therapist and district nurse become important, especially to those who have no one else to share their successes or discuss their worries. If your GP is not sympathetic, you or your family should search for a replacement, because it is essential that all of you should have confidence in your medical adviser. One recovering patient raised another point. She felt insecure and inadequate when she did not conform to what she termed the 'time signposts' suggested by doctors and others. Told that she should have progressed faster she felt threatened by what she felt was being judged against vague guidelines. Again it seems important how such goals are suggested. Minor, realistic targets can be a challenge, but any targets set in a negative way – you will not be able to do this, or you cannot expect to do this for a long time – can be a real deterrent. One of the worst of these is to be told that after a certain time has passed you cannot expect further improvement. Sadly this is a common experience, and one that has to be challenged.

The attitude of friends and family can also affect the patient. Some people made it clear that they thought that the stroke was basically the end for me – the end of my working life and usefulness at least. This of course is what the general perception of a stroke patient is and in turn affects how some people react to you thereafter. It is almost the same as a bereavement. I have heard others recount how acquaintances cross over the road rather than meet them face to face because they do not know what to say. You can see it in the faces of people in shops and restaurants and occasionally overhear comments. Anyone who has used a wheelchair knows this kind of thing only too well. It also affects how others offer help. Many people are afraid of long term commitment. They would rush to visit and help a patient with a broken leg, but a stroke patient – that is an open-ended commitment, and let us be honest, most people today lead rushed lives. It is when you return home that visits from friends become so important. It is then that you could easily begin to feel isolated and lonely, especially if you live alone.

When first venturing out and about acquaintances can, inadvertently, be a real menace. You need all your attention so as not to trip on uneven surfaces. To turn round, or even look up, can be quite dangerous at that stage. Yet acquaintances rush up from all directions and ask you whatever you have done to yourself. Worse still they may insist on taking your arm, which immediately throws you off balance. Then there are the constant explanations and the look of shock and embarrassment on the faces of people who expected to hear of a broken bone or a hip replacement, and instead hear of a stroke.

Attitudes to walking aids

Aids to mobility are there to be used when essential, but it is vital not to become dependent on any one longer than strictly necessary. It is a big step to leave the safety of the wheelchair and take your first steps from living room to the kitchen, leaning on a stick. It is real progress, a significant triumph and the first judgement to make between support and safety. The next step may be for how long a leg splint may be either needed or even desirable, or built up shoes or even a stick. Ideally the decision should be taken jointly by patient and physiotherapist, but the real situation is often far from ideal. It is at such a time, as Jane Cast (page 67) points out, that the patient is likely to be out of contact with therapists, just when they could do with sound advice and encouragement. The decision of when to stop depending on a walking aid is just as important as having advice earlier on about the availability of suitable aids. In the end the final decision will be taken by the patients in the privacy of their own home, balancing safety against a gradual return to normality. Much may once more depend on the attitude of those around them, family and friends – either encouraging them to take a calculated risk and move on, or worrying too much about safety and holding them back.

A personal note

It soon became apparent that my cheerful demeanour confused people. Some, like my hospital physiotherapists, approved of it and made use of the fact that I was not sunk in depression. Many people underestimated the severity of my disabilities, and that was reflected back on the way I thought. That was no bad thing at the time, though perhaps later on it was a bit of a disadvantage when I may have been judged as being less in need of help than I was. Then there were those who seemed annoyed by my optimism, and preferred to try and disillusion me. Whatever other people thought, I could not and would not have changed my reactions to the initial effects of the stroke. Privately, I was by no means always as cheerful as I appeared in public, and had some pretty black moments as I realised the implications. Somehow there did not seem to be any alternative but to appear cheerful and positive. I had learned long ago from visiting elderly relatives, how easy it is to deter visitors by detailing one's woes. Anyhow, to have given in to the many problems that still existed would not only have blighted my life but my husband's as well.

In retrospect, after two years, it is more annoying now that all the novelty has worn off. I may be much further along the path to recovery but, whereas I would have once accepted it, I now get more frustrated by my slowness and clumsiness, not less. Tiredness limits my activities, but I am constantly reminded of the effects of adrenalin (though suppressed by medication). When I really want to do something I often find it becomes possible to do it, though I may pay for it in tiredness the next day or so. When I suddenly find myself in a challenging situation I may find, to my surprise, that it is possible to meet that challenge. That confirms my feeling that you do not necessarily reach a plateau, you can always push yourself or be pushed further forward.

Progress and suggestions

THREE YEARS ON and the perspective shifts again. To the outsider there may be little improvement in my condition when they see me out of my home environment. To those who have not seen me since my stroke there is still the same reaction of shock and pity, but to me, and to those nearest to me, it is a different matter. Measured against some point − what I could do last year at the same time, or just last time I visited a certain place, it is obvious how much difference there is. I am no longer worried to go up a few steps without the support of a rail or banister. I can manage soft sand on the beach and get into the ocean (provided it is not too rough), a feat that was impossible last summer.

My foot seldom clumps up in panic at a bump in the path, and the nightly cramps improve slowly. It may be that I have more stamina rather than improved gait, or even that I am more relaxed and confident. I still need to concentrate on my walking when in unfamiliar surroundings and crowded pavements are still a bit of a problem. My arm is stronger and hand function is much improved from the days when I could grasp objects but had difficulty in releasing my grip − just like a baby. It is usage rather than any specific exercise that has accomplished this. Gadgets like an electric tin-opener and toothbrush have helped make some jobs easier. I am still a rather messy eater, but probably no one would notice other than myself these days.

There are even some positive improvements. My left hand was always pretty useless, but now I have become more ambidextrous. I used to speak too fast, now I am much slower which many people tell me is a great advantage. In the same way organisational powers have sharpened to devise strategies to utilise limited energy. So, in addition to speech, thinking and writing (by computer) have become better organised and perhaps deeper.

I have a greater understanding of the children with handwriting problems, dyspraxic and other, that I still see as part of my work in that field. I now know what it feels like to be able to write a few words slowly and moderately legibly, yet not be able to write anything fast. I can imagine how frustrating it must be to be criticised, and can say from experience that exercises might be counterproductive, causing more tension and deteriorating movement. I have experienced the puzzling phenomenum of the reversal of numbers. For quite a while a 6 came out when a 9 was called for and vice versa, and I was unable to take down a telephone number without several other inexplicable mistakes. Those are more reminders of the strange workings of the brain. Such problems sometimes solve themselves and, sadly, sometimes do not.

From reading this you may get the impression that I spend my time analysing my situation. Far from it, I am very lucky. The computer has enabled me to carry on my main occupation of writing books and articles on a variety of subjects. I even manage to do a certain amount of lecturing, and still see a procession of children (and a few adults) with literacy problems. As well as that I design typefaces that are meant for educational purposes and to be extra legible on the computer screen. Mentally, I am kept pretty busy and I cannot complain that life is dull – only sometimes rather tiring.

The minutiae of daily life, such as shopping, cooking and

gardening take up rather more of my time than they would have done before the stroke, and I need more help with larger household tasks which I still find awkward. It is only leisure activities that are more limited through lack of mobility, as I no longer drive more than short distances, but that is not too much of a deprivation.

Small occurrences like catching flu, can still set me back and my limited efforts at handwriting (usually confined to addressing envelopes) demonstrate only too clearly when I am having a bad day. I have found that letting myself go too long without food is a mistake. Hunger seems to have as bad an effect on memory and movement as over-tiredness. Sudden thirst also needs attention, but that is not too difficult. It means keeping a bottle of water nearby when I am away from home.

Occasionally some part of me still reveals weakness or a need to be more flexible; then it is an interesting challenge to devise some exercise at home or in the swimming pool. It may not be what a therapist would recommend but usually works. The time scale may have changed but the truth is undeniable. Improvement is taking place all the time and shows no sign of reaching a plateau (a term I became conversant with early on in my convalescence).

Unexpected things remained problematic and there are times when I have had to force myself forwards. It was strangely difficult, for instance, to regain enough confidence to drive myself, long after I was judged capable of the task. It was all too easy to find some excuse why not to take the challenge, risk, or whatever you might call it. I am even more convinced now, than I was when this all began, that the battle for the mind of a patient – at any stage – is as vital as the battle for, or what may be seen as the emphasis on, the body. There is a compulsion to talk about all this, not only to confound those who declared that there would be a time limit on improvement, but to try and change the public perception of the condition.

Compiling this book has made me realise how much information I have accumulated in these last three years. At the same time it shows how little I knew about how certain parts of the body work or of the terminology of stroke rehabilitation. For example, at a vulnerable stage I was confronted by: 'Of course you trip and stub your toes, it is the result of drop foot'. How was I to know what drop foot was? I knew a bit about hands but legs and feet were outside my experience. The phrases that professionals use must seem common place to them but to patients they add to the confusion. Explanation and information can take away much of the fear and worry, and help you to understand what you can do to help yourself. Is it too much to ask for?

Inevitably, I wonder how much further on I would be by now if more and better therapy had been available, or whether my self-help methods have been just as successful. I have been fortunate, however, in other ways. The expertise and advice (if not actual therapy) of colleagues with whom I had worked earlier on, and people I became involved with by sheer luck, has had a profound effect on my recovery. I cannot recommend this self-help therapy unreservedly. It has had a reasonable outcome for me, has contributed to a kind of pride in my own achievement, and was essential as there was no provision for ongoing rehabilitation in my area, not even in the private sector. I have, however, met some people, just as determined as I was, who have not had such successful outcomes.

As I talk to more and more people I realise how lucky I have been not to have suffered any intellectual impairment, as so much has depended on my being able to plan any action in advance. It must be so much harder when you cannot communicate. Many others tell me that they suffer pain as a result of their stroke. Where there is residual pain after several years it seems even more reprehensible when they report that they have had no help.

Where can people obtain meaningful literature? If they go to their public library there is no guarantee that what they find will be appropriate or up to date. Jane Cast (see page 65) went to investigate what was available at her local library and was unhappy to find only something over ten years old, that recommended practices that she considered out of date and inadequate. A book that would be useful is *Stroke at our Fingertips* by Dr A Rudd, P Irwin and B Penhale, published in 2000 by Class Publishing. It covers all aspects of life after stroke.

The Stroke Association, the only national charity concerned solely with stroke, has a comprehensive list of their own pamphlets and publications. Many people today would turn to the internet to find out more about stroke. There they will find a vast amount of up-to-date information. It is only necessary to remember that there is no censorship on the internet and it is prudent to check any medical suggestions with your doctor before acting on them.

Although it is vital that comprehensive information should be widely available, it must add to the frustration, even desperation, of patients and carers to read of management plans, intensive speech therapy, pain clinics or other assistance, when none is offered locally. The difference between what appears in the literature as the right way forward, and what is actually available country-wide is only too clear to many of us. With the best of intentions, I understand that it will be a long time before enough trained personnel will be available to implement the proposals that are now being put forward.

Suggestions

Strokes affect people in such different ways. I realise the limitations of my own experience and therefore the precise relevance of it to any other patient. I was too old for it to affect my career, yet young enough for me to have the energy to fight the effects. On the whole my damage was limited to motor functions, and I had the support of a caring husband. Certain general suggestions, however, can be made from the view of a patient. The best advice that I was given was offered about a month after my stroke. It came from a young, newly qualified physiotherapist. 'You will be improving for the rest of your life' she said. I was not willing to accept it at the time, with its depressing implication of my not being fully recovered for the rest of my life.

Now I look at it in a different light. A certain amount of long term damage is now obvious, and that message is a message of hope and not the opposite. To further that improvement the best advice I can think of is to consider any action that is tiring or awkward to perform as therapy. I recently met a lady who had not recovered full use of her arm after nearly five years. Isolated, without treatment, she said it was too tiring to use her right arm so she did not do so. I told her of my way of dealing with the same problem – months of struggling to hang out the washing (aided by making the arm work hard while swimming) managed to strengthen it. At first you may feel sick and dizzy with effort, later on only very tired, but it works in the end. You have to listen to your body and recognise the need to give in to weariness. Never be ashamed of having a rest in the afternoon, or even in the morning if you feel you need it, (in the early days, the effort of getting dressed and eating breakfast was enough to make me want to retire to a comfortable sofa and have a short sleep). However, I am not aware that pushing yourself to the edge of tiredness from time to time in order to improve function does much harm. I only hope it was the correct advice for her.

It follows that with this attitude there is a need to ignore any suggested cut-off dates for further improvement. How often I heard 'You will make the most rapid recovery in the first few weeks', with the implication that as I was still in a wheelchair after two months the next stages would be slower and less successful. Then, after another two months – 'You can do almost all you need, you do not require any more therapy', indeed a suggestion that too much therapy was harmful. If I had believed that I might have given up trying there and then. Next, someone whose judgement I respect, when admiring how far I had progressed in the first year gave what was meant to be kindly advice – 'You cannot expect much more improvement after a year'. Further comments, equally kindly meant, express pleasure and astonishment that I am still so patently improving after three years. This would not come as a surprise if only attitudes could be more positive.

As I meet more people I hear the same story. One particular case of a young teenager worried me. He was more than eighteen months on in his recovery and had made good progress. He was determined and very brave – but worried. He had been told by his doctor not to expect any further progress after two years. He knew that he would not have adequate hand function, in particular, by the approaching deadline. It was obvious with his determination that the prognosis would be proven wrong, but what a cruel burden and unnecessary worry for a young boy and his parents. Others report being told that they will be confined to a wheelchair for life, when it has proved patently untrue.

Everyone needs hope, yet few people seem to be given

the advice that the more they exert themselves the better their progress will be – and that they will continue to improve as long as they persevere. Progress may not be so dramatic later on, or so noticeable to others, but everyone should be encouraged to rejoice in how they are recovering even (or perhaps particularly) when it is happening slowly.

Finding new occupations

It is important to find interesting occupations that are within the capabilities of the person recovering. Many older people (or their relatives) have reported how distressed they were at being unable to continue with their usual leisure activities, such a sewing or other craft work. It is not only a feeling of uselessness that this engenders, but of boredom and does nothing to alleviate depression. Finding something suitable probably puts one more burden on carers and they may need to exercise considerable imagination (and perhaps tact as well).

I have developed a strategy that works for me when going through a bad patch. To motivate myself to get up and start the day, I think of a small task or pleasurable occupation that I would be capable of doing. It sounds rather trite, but it usually stops me from thinking of all the things I cannot do.

Some of the occupations in day centres seem rather patronising and unimaginative when offered to intelligent adults. Because you are physically disabled, temporarily or permanently, does not mean that your intellect has been affected. Painting by numbers might keep patients 'occupied' but if paints were available as well as plenty of bowls of flowers around, as I once witnessed, some people might have been offered the option of something freer and more challenging. I am probably being unfair, but this kind of incident makes me cringe. As a patient you are vulnerable in many different ways. A patient would be unlikely to complain about such a trivial matter as their intelligence being underestimated. It would be one more slight indignity to be borne among many worse. But such occurrences, added together, chip away at a person's spirit and self-confidence. It would, I suppose, boil down to the competence and willingness to go that one step further by an individual therapist,

The following example suggests that you never can foresee what will succeed and what unusual benefits a new activity might bring. In a book by American artist Barbara Roberts entitled *Catie Learns to Draw*, an interesting view is put forward. She maintains that, instead of trying to attempt something that the patients did expertly before the stroke, they should be encouraged to start new activities where there would be no negative comparison to make. Roberts illustrated some amazing work undertaken under her tuition by a stroke patient, who had never attempted any art work before. She used a technique where the drawing is done almost entirely without looking at the work in progress. What is more extraordinary is that she reports that Catie had a slight 'neglect' on her left side (see page 142) and needed constant prompting to look left. The art therapy seems to have helped her to overcome some of that aspect of her disability as well as giving her immense satisfaction and, as Roberts reports, a feeling of self-worth again.

Barbara Roberts was first and foremost an artist, not a therapist, which makes her contribution even more interesting. Since writing of Catie's case she has been drawn to helping more stroke patients, and talks of the incredible satisfaction that she has found in putting her skills to this usage. She reports two results which merit serious consideration. One is that all the patients seem to produce a very similar style of work; furthermore others who displayed a neglect of one side or the other improved after working with her technique.

An occupational therapist suggested that we need not think of art therapy solely in terms of painting. She felt that a more tangible and perhaps less threatening craft such as pottery might induce as immediate a sense of achievement, and be just as confidence-building. Moreover, the creating of a three dimensional piece, however simple, involves planning sequencing and other beneficial strategies. There is plenty of room for both points of view. However, Barbara Roberts' work reinforces my feelings that quite often people from a completely different field can use their special skills to benefit patients and make discoveries in ways that conventionally trained therapists would not, or could not attempt.

Perhaps I should mention here that I also went to art school and first worked as a designer and letterer, which is why I am particularly intertested in this aspect of therapy. I taught and wrote about those subjects before getting involved in the educational and medical aspects of hand-writing. Finally, I turned to mainly research orientated work.

The late Sir Harry Secombe made a short television programme about his recovery from a stroke. There was a brief mention in it of music therapy, though more as a muscle strengthening activity for a man who had a classical operatic training than for pleasure. It carried the same implicit message as Barbara Roberts: that, at a vulnerable stage of recovery, it might not always be a good idea to allow comparisons between pre-stroke expertise and post-stroke capability. Watching this film – and noting the standard of therapy he was receiving – reminded me of my own resolution should I suffer a second stroke. I would gratefully accept any in-patient treatment provided by the National Health Service but would try to follow that up with a stay in one of the private rehabilitation facilities that give intensive integrated therapy.

I would make a special plea here for those who have lost the power to speak – those suffering from aphasia. There are many, like the patient mentioned on page.17, who are not being recognised as able to communicate but are quite capable of writing when given the opportunity. I met another such case when I was in hospital but could not intervene except by telling his wife what I had observed and hoping that someone would follow it up. Just recently I heard of a man who could neither speak coherently nor write, but managed to communicate his thoughts clearly by means of detailed drawings. An article in The Times on 10 July 2001 discussed the problem of aphasia. Part of its message was that there is hope and that there are several alternative ways of communication. A statement from the Connect centre in Borough, South London (website: www.connect.org.uk) reported: 'Most people who attend Connect's centre arrive hoping to to get their speech back. Mainly, however, the aim has to be to help them to make the most of other forms of communication, such as drawing, intonation, facial expression or gesture. We aim to help people to understand how their lives have changed.'

It may seem inappropriate to some patients that I should discuss sporting activities or even recreation. Richard Lockwood makes a case for this in Recreation and Disability in Australia: 'For people with disability (and this obviously applies to stroke patients among many others) recreation has been an elusive goal. With so much emphasis on planned rehabilitation the creativity and joy derived from participation has often been overridden by management constraints'. As for sport you only have to look at the paralympics to see what severely handicapped athletes can achieve. I am not suggesting anything as dramatic as that. I remember seeing sports therapy in action in Beijing, where wheelchair-bound stroke patients were being encouraged to participate in basket ball games. In our district hospital's occupational therapy unit patients enjoyed playing darts, which had the added advantage of improving co-ordination and balance. Swimming has been my preferred activity, starting with all too brief sessions in a hydrotherapy pool, then other public pools and finally the ocean. Swimming was both excellent therapy and a pleasure. I am still not very elegant in the water, but then I never was before my stroke.

Finally, the computer provides a multitude of new opportunities for leisure and learning for all ages, as well as enabling a housebound patient to communicate with the outside world. I feel that there will be a gap in the market for challenging computer games for older people as more housebound adults depend on their computer to entertain, as well as to broaden their horizons. As the generation who use computers every day for work and recreation begin to form a larger part of older patients – whether affected from stroke or other conditions – they, quite rightly, will expect their needs to be addressed.

Stroke clubs and self-help groups

There is a desperate need to help alleviate the loneliness of many patients whose lives have become limited through loss of mobility. One way would be to start stroke clubs in the many districts where none are available. We became involved in trying to start such a group in our locality where the health authority no longer supports one. Such a group must take account of the needs of that specific community, so our first objective when we had found a suitable location, would be to set up an inaugural meeting, after publicising our intention as widely as possible. Something that could provide specialist advice, or even therapy would be ideal. Our priority was to identify the need, get something small started, then let it grow of its own accord. We have met with a few problems and have yet to succeed.

A self-help group can function at several levels, even where it is not able to provide any actual therapy. At the most basic it can provide a meeting place for patients to discuss their problems and exchange ideas. It can provide simple facilities for leisure, appropriate for those who attend. This might break down some of the feeling of isolation that many of those experience when recovering from a stroke. Helping with the organisation of such a group might add to patients' self-esteem and bring back meaning into lonely lives. At the same time a regular meeting might provide a valuable hour of freedom for carers – unless they would prefer to meet others in the same predicament and share some of their concerns.

The Stroke Association (www.stroke.org.uk) keeps a list of all affiliated stroke clubs, and more information can be obtained from their regional offices .

Different age groups have different needs. An example of what can be done can be seen in the activities of the organisation Different Strokes (see page 127) who have set up exercise groups for younger people around the country.

Alternatives

Whether a certain amount of out-patient therapy is available or not, helpful and sometimes unorthodox advice can often be gleaned from other people along the way. Some of the most useful tips I have had have come from unexpected sources. An elderly nun in hospital gave me the only help I received for dealing with a stiff, lopsided mouth. It was to try to whistle. It took a long time but eventually it worked. On holiday a couple of years later a nurse noticed my foot clumping on the cold stones as I tried to get into the swimming pool. 'Try clenching and unclenching your toes', she said – another exercise that seemed impossible at first, but helped in the end. About the same time, my daughter, who has been on the receiving end of some interesting alternative therapies, tried stimulating the nerve endings on my toes. These extremities were the last to respond to my attempts to make contact (see page 22) She was as surprised as I was when they responded with the quiver that, with perseverance, develops into controlled movement.

Alternative therapies such as aromatherapy, reflexology, and any of the many relaxation techniques might help. Different massages, tried out on my travels abroad, were particularly helpful, but I was never long enough in one place to discover whether they would have a lasting effect. I remember, some years ago, seeing a whole ward of patients in a rehabilitation hospital in Beijing undergoing acupuncture. Research is currently being undertaken in this country to determine how effective this treatment is (see page 155). It did not help me, but that was hardly a fair test as the practitioner admitted that she was just learning the technique. Also, acupuncture is probably most effective soon after a stroke, and I only tried it some two years later.

We are all, however, dependent on what is available locally. It seems to me that sensitive practitioners who will use their knowledge to adapt their techniques to your specific problem are just as important as the particular therapy itself. If I had to make a judgement I would think a mix of traditional and eastern therapies might be the perfect answer. All that it is sensible to say is that you should not expect miracles. You should try not to become too dependent on anything or anyone. That is the way to disillusionment and even despair when something or someone does not live up to expectations. Quite recently I heard of a patient who had pinned his hopes on a leg splint to help him walk again. When this failed he sank deeper into depression and gave up hope of ever becoming mobile.

An alternative, but not unorthodox, way of dealing with rehabilitation is what might be termed integrated therapy. This suggests that multi-disciplinary therapists, or at least those who have the skills and will to cross professional barriers, might be most successful. A pioneering private clinic that employs integrated therapy described their methods this way: 'Staff are skilled in each other's jobs to ensure patients are constantly stimulated. Physiotherapists talk to patients, speech therapists help them to move'.

Patients, once back in the community, in addition to their physical management deserve better understanding of what, for want of a better term, are their psychological needs. There needs to be informed encouragement from everyone concerned to assist individuals to maximise their recovery, whatever the local provision of therapy may be.

Part 2

DIFFERENT PERSPECTIVES

The part played by the contributors

OST OF THOSE who have contributed to the second part of this book are part of my own story of recovery and discovery. The account starts with my attempts to find a walking aid to replace the ill-fitting splint that came out of a cupboard in hospital, and was only meant as a temporary safety measure. I felt it was impeding rather than aiding my progress. Enquiries led me to the orthotist at the district hospital the day my original physiotherapist (see page 24) was asking for volunteers to take part in a training day to be run by the team from Salisbury on the use of the Odstock Dropped Foot Stimulator (ODFS). One thing led to another and a couple of months later I was accepted on the programme described by Paul Taylor and Jane Burridge on page 72.

To be part of a research project is, in itself, an enormous boost to any patient's morale. To meet people whose expertise is so evident gives you hope, apart from the obvious practical consequences. The first trial with the ODFS at Salisbury Hospital showed a dramatic improvement in my walking speed. However, I had the feeling that it would not be good for me if the device took over the act of lifting my dropped foot all the time. (It was only at Salisbury that the term 'drop-foot' was finally explained to me.) It was agreed that I should use the device only half of the time, even though at that time there was no evidence that there was a carry-over effect (i.e. that it would help my muscles to learn to do the job themselves). I always felt, however, that an echo remained to activate those muscles for an instant, after the switch was turned off. It is difficult to separate the effects of the ODFS in retraining my leg to help itself, and the other factors involved. Using the device reminded me of how it felt to walk naturally again and helped to lengthen my stride from the typical short, tentative steps of the stroke patient. Then a growing confidence in my ability to move without tripping over at each step encouraged more walking. All this contributed, over a period of about a year, to the gradual strengthening of my whole leg until it seemed time to make it do its own work. I am convinced that the Odstock Dropped Foot Stimulator contributed considerably to the speed of my recovery, although I cannot claim to have contributed much to research in return. However, it was interesting to learn that now the opinion is that patients should not use the device full time, to avoid the problem of becoming overdependent on it.

A gait analysis

The next episode took place in Australia. For many years we have spent part of the (northern) winter in Perth and I have had friendly contact with the department of Human Movement in the University of Western Australia. Some nine months after my stroke we took the risk of keeping to our usual habit, only to find that flying half way around the world was considerably easier than taking a commuter train from our local station to London. You are given a wheelchair (which is still necessary because of the distance in airports) and looked after at every stage of the journey.

I took my equipment to the department to show it off, and was rewarded by an offer to do a comparative gait analysis with and without the FES (Functional Electrical Stimulation).

This test consists of fixing markers on strategic points of my body and limbs so that they appear on the computer, allowing a complete picture of my movements. Speed, force and cadence were among the factors measured. Although I did not appreciate it at the time, reading it again now I can see how many details it revealed – the weakness of my knee and upper leg that I eventually realised myself, and used an inexpensive pedal machine to strengthen, and the need to lengthen my stride that still needs more work today – and much more.

Incidentally, on the same day as the gait analysis another vital service was offered. Curtin University runs a driving assessment centre fully equipped with simulators and other testing equipment. At that time I was worried that, in order to keep my licence from being taken away, there was a test to be taken on returning home. This centre provided an opportunity to find out how I was likely to perform, away from the tension of an actual test situation. It pinpointed what aspects needed to improve and was a great relief. Such centres are also available throughout Great Britain.

Practical therapy at last

Pete Hamer and David Lloyd's detailed gait analysis awaited me on our return to England, but it was more than six months later before Jane Cast (see page 65) could interpret it properly for me. She is an experienced community neuro-physiotherapist and was fully occupied at that time working locally for Cheshire Homes. Like my Australian friends, she was shocked by the condition that I had been left in. She could not offer me intensive therapy and rather doubted whether I would, by myself, be able to correct the bent posture and awkward gait that I had adopted. She gave a detailed explanation of my condition and the precise purpose of each of the exercises she prescribed. This, combined with my own shock at realising how bad I had let my whole situation become, made me discipline myself to keep to a fairly rigid regime. For the first time I found how satisfying systematic exercise was, and how quickly results could be seen. It took only three informal visits over a period of perhaps six weeks to get me upright, and transferring my weight properly from one foot to another.

There are several conclusions to draw from this from the patient's angle:

1. Therapists cannot take it for granted that a positive reply means that a patient understands all that they are being told, for example that they understand terms such as tone, or that the patients, when optimists, are really as far recovered as they appear.

2. How easy it is and how dangerous to get the balance wrong between regaining function and learning good movement.

3. How difficult it is for people to realise when they are not upright with their weight evenly balanced, or to work out quite obvious strategies that would benefit them.

4. How difficult it is to self-correct without guidance, but how quickly results can come from just a little clear expert advice.

5. How, with expert help, it is never too late to retrain and improve

Perhaps we have both helped each other, because the speed with which her exercise regime changed my life has encouraged her to take on more long-term, neglected patients.

Jane has found the same kind of results which she reports in her section starting on page 65. I learned that it is the precise description of how an exercise should be carried out, and what its purpose is, allied to the placing of the body correctly so that you can feel what is correct, that allows you to help yourself. The attitude of the therapist makes a huge difference. He or she needs to show a difficult mix of positive encouragement and firmness. Above all the patient needs to feel that therapists know what they are doing and that they really care about achieving a result. There must be a mutual respect, with the patient's views and wishes taken into account. Exercises insufficiently explained and given too early, before people have the strength to do them properly, may cause them to lose faith in exercise altogether. The episode of the gait analysis emphasised how difficult it is to self-correct, and how essential an expert intervention is, irrespective of the stage of recovery.

Jane is just starting her new job as Stroke Care Co-ordinator, across South West Kent Primary Care Trust. This includes collecting relevant data, surveying existing local services to see how they can be improved and looking at examples of good practice in other trusts. These activities should be taking place in health authorities country-wide in conjunction with the National Service Framework (NFS) for Older People. (see page 118) and the clinical guidelines of the Royal College of Physicians .

Occupational therapy

I had little personal experience of good practice in occu-pational therapy during my recovery, although the safety equipment recommended and demonstrated by the OT department helped me considerably on my return home. The shower seat was particularly successful and I still use it.

The therapy that was provided might have been sufficient for the very elderly who needed only the most basic skills in the home, but lacked understanding of anyone needing any more. I am not being critical of the teaching of essential daily living skills and realise that they are very important, particularly for patients who will be living alone. I am making a plea for a bit more thought about individual needs. Having once, at an earlier stage of my professional life, fought for signature writing to be included as a daily living skill, it seems to me that there now needs to be further advances in that area, to equip patients for a fuller and more satisfying life once they are back in their own homes.

My first priority, admittedly rather unusual, was assurance that I would be able to manipulate a keyboard one-handed. A request to try that instead of tea making was met with incredulity. Yet computers play such a vital part in most people's lives, surely it is time to consider them more seriously. Apart from the fact that many disabled people may become dependent on computers to communicate, even to do their daily shopping, the use of a keyboard is excellent therapy (with instant feedback in terms of increasing accuracy, just like handwriting). It may be difficult for older therapists to appreciate how widely and naturally their patients will have used computers. They (the therapists) may feel threatened by something they do not wholly understand. Patients may also need guidance about more specialised technology to help them in their new life (or at least information as to where to access this).

I am aware that there is an acute shortage of occupational therapists in our part of the world and that, in all fairness, with constant staff changes the whole ethos of a department can alter considerably over a period of time.

Speech and language therapy

I did not have, or witness, any speech and language therapy, although the need for a speech therapist in the rehabilitation unit was obvious. It was by chance that I met Deborah Harding (see page 84), when our train to London was delayed one morning, and we soon discovered our mutual interest. A Registered Member of the Royal College of Speech and Language Therapists she has practised as a speech and language therapist in the field of adult neuro-rehabilitation, having first completed an M.Sc. in Cognitive Neuro-psychology at the University of London. She has published papers in the area of cognitive neuro-psychological approaches to aphasia therapy, as well as writing on broader service delivery issues. She currently manages a multi-disciplinary team at West Kent Neuro-rehabilitation Unit. A member of the British Aphasiology Society, she served for six years as Secretary to the Society.

Bobath technique

The link with the article by Dr Mayston (see page 79) on the Bobath technique dates back to my early days in hospital. One of the young physiotherapists had returned from an advanced Bobath course. The techniques she had learned were an immediate advance, felt by patients and the others who gathered round to learn. How I agree with these sentences from the Bobath concept (see page 80), on the part motivation also plays when being set and achieving meaningful and relevant goals:

'While it was thought that teaching people normal movement patterns and postural reactions would automatically lead to the performance of functional tasks, it is now known that the activity of the CNS is task dependent (Flament et al, 1993 and Ehrsson, et al 2000). Therefore it is essential that therapists work with clients to achieve goals that are relevant to their lives, and not goals decided for them by therapists.'

Cognitive therapy and doctors' attitudes

I contacted Kit Malia and Anne Brannagan after hearing their presentation at the 2001 annual conference of Different Strokes. So little is known about their subject that their contribution is particularly valuable. Kit Malia, with a research degree in neuro-psychology, is the only certified Cognitive Rehabilitation Therapist in the UK (via the Society for Cognitive Rehabilitation, USA). He has worked for over a decade with adults who have acquired neurological injuries in the Defence Services Rehabilitation Centre, Headley Court. Anne Brannagan is the senior Neurological Occupational Therapist and the deputy coordinator of the Neurological Rehabilitation team at Headley Court.

Professor McLellan, as Great Britain's first professor of rehabilitation, needs no introduction to anyone in the field. I was fortunate to visit his department in Southampton several years before my stroke. His sensitive contribution describes the changing attitudes of doctors as they are trained in rehabilitation medicine. One matter he stresses is that: 'While two strokes may appear much the same, two people with strokes never are, and that the attributes and objectives of the person who has a stroke are crucial elements in negotiating what rehabilitation should aim at, and what form it should take.'

It seems that those who have contributed to this part of the book share many similar views.

CHAPTER 6

Physiotherapy: the importance of a physical management plan

JANE CAST

As a physiotherapist with an interest in neurology, particularly the issues arising from those with a long term disability, the importance of an ongoing management plan in their daily lives has become apparent to me. It is devastating to see someone who has suffered from a stroke, told the diagnosis, admitted to hospital for varying amounts of rehabilitation, then literally cast into the community and left to get on with it. There is so much ongoing rehabilitation that could help people to reach their full potential, yet it seems there is a cut-off point when everyone assumes that there is nothing more that can be done. People are left wondering why no one shows any more interest. They feel entirely on their own with no further guidance as to what they might achieve.

Treating neurological patients in the community has revealed how little rehabilitation can be offered to those in certain areas of the country. People who wish to try and improve their physical capabilities generally have no plan of action once they get back home. Out-patient or community physiotherapy may be arranged for a short time only. If not, it may be assumed that they will continue to improve without further assistance and direction. This also means that some will deteriorate with no further input and possibly return back to the hospital. An unnecessary pattern of crisis management may then develop. This reminds me of a patient who had a mild stroke and was not judged to need any physiotherapy on discharge from hospital. When she was seen a few years later after several falls and failing to cope at home the results of this neglect were apparent. One-sided, with significant balance problems and the inability to transfer weight successfully, she needed much more intensive treatment to overcome these acquired disabilities.

People often do not realise how their condition has changed. When questioned about what exercises they are doing they may reply: 'The ones shown in hospital' – even if this was several years after! Aids given out initially may now no longer be needed. Patients have no guidelines to follow and fear a deterioration if they change anything. It could be that the complete opposite is true for some. The body may be allowed to recruit more normal movement patterns when an aid is withdrawn. With ongoing recovery people deserve more understanding of how to manage their condition. They need to understand how modifying their efforts and using normal patterns of movement will help to promote further recovery.

Everyone should realise that patients can continue to improve long after their stroke. I recently visited a patient some two years after his stroke. Without ongoing treatment he was confined to a wheelchair. The complicating factor was his height; he was six foot four. He had mastered transfers but nobody had had the courage to try to get him to walk. We made it a challenge and worked out a friendly 'contract', allowing him, initially, to set the timescale. Intermediate goals were the next stage, proving the patient's own estimate to have been highly pessimistic. He is still making good progress towards walking.

Physiotherapy does not need to be daily, weekly or even monthly, however, there should be somebody involved who has a particular interest in neurology. These are the people best able to assess and re-assess each individual's needs. They can give patients new goals, set new programmes, explore new challenges as well as offer patients the motivation and support they need to believe they can become more functionally independent. This, for most people, is their aim, but a lack of specialised physiotherapists can make accessing their service difficult.

Ongoing help

A stroke comes as a devastating event and initially people are unable to fully appreciate the extent of the damage. That realisation will not come until a much later stage. It is important that at this point they receive informed, positive help to look to the future. An encouraging attitude can help to alleviate depression and combat the fear that this is how they are destined to live the rest of their lives. People need informed help to enable them to focus on what they are trying to achieve and to analyse how best to approach the task. This can be neglected in hospital, as time constraints are very difficult.

Stroke management at home, once they are medically stable and able to transfer, can offer advantages. They are in a familiar environment so it is easier to identify more realistic goals. Patients start to understand how they can take more responsibility for their own recovery. Working at home allows simple exercises to be incorporated into daily activities. In this way the constant reinforcement of exercises and positioning throughout the day has a long lasting beneficial effect – as long as they are done correctly. The patient can be given an uninterrupted one-to-one session, which is often not possible in a busy out-patient department or ward. Patients may also feel more at ease to express their worries and identify more specific activities that are a problem in their home environment. These can then be assessed and a plan of action implemented to either improve or alter their activity.

The physiotherapist plays an important role in educating people about the potential they have and then encouraging them to reach out to achieve goals that otherwise they might have thought impossible. Positive feedback can only help to further their drive and desire to make more effort themselves. The more they achieve the more likely they are to want to do more. Lack of input or a challenge can lead to deterioration, low morale and poor outcome. It is amazing how a few simple words of advice can help to move somebody on to the next stage.

Another function of a physiotherapist is multidisciplinary working and liaison to ensure that all the patient's needs are adequately met. The importance of the role of the carer should also be considered; he or she can make a huge difference. An enthusiastic new carer gave Mary a new lease of life fifteen years after her stroke. Spending time with her, showing her a few simple positions, how to stretch and involve her hand in daily exercises allowed Mary to move her fingers at long last. For therapists and carers alike it is extremely satisfying to work with those in the community whose needs have been neglected, and to give them new hope. A team approach should enable patients to achieve independence in many aspects of life.

The benefits of talking to professionals cannot be underestimated. They have the vital experience and knowledge of appropriate treatments, aids and adaptations. An ongoing physical management plan can be developed following discussion and assessment, looking at a broad spectrum of activities. This should be reviewed at regular intervals and adjusted as necessary. Any plan needs to take into account what is available in the locality but should be tailored to suit each individual's need. The emphasis should be on appropriate advice, education and treatment. Some form of supervision will be required to ensure that the plan is being followed correctly and its goals fulfilled.

Areas that are often neglected

Through working with a broad spectrum of neurological patients it is possible to observe certain common areas of neglect that frequently occur. This can lead to reduced functional ability, unnecessary pain and weakness in joints and muscles, which in turn prevent patients from developing their full physical potential.

The concept of normal movement sequences, tone and balance are key factors around which stroke recovery and rehabilitation are based. It is therefore vital that the patients are given time for a detailed explanation of what they are trying to achieve while the therapists are working with them to facilitate the movement. If patients and carers appreciate what they are aiming at, or at least what they are expected to do, they are far more likely to succeed. This can also prevent the development of a series of secondary complications, through misunderstanding the complex physical effects of the stroke.

The emphasis on rehabilitation can often be on getting the patient to transfer and walk in order to be able to return home. This may result in a neglected arm and hand. In the meantime patients can become increasingly skilled at managing all activities one handed and so the full potential of the affected one is never developed.

The arm can be a source of many problems. Patients frequently experience loss of movement – and therefore loss of function – as well as varying degrees of pain. It can be a long and gradual process awaiting any return of active movement in the arm. Meanwhile, much can be done to encourage patients to adopt an appropriate management plan. This should ensure that they do not lose vital ranges of movement, and also should promote a bilateral approach.

The positioning of the arm, both in bed and sitting in the chair, is important. This is in order to normalise tone or to protect an arm with low tone. It is also relevant when there is loss of sensation and neglect. Joints should be kept as mobile as possible and handled very carefully. Pain, contractures, subluxation of the shoulder, loss of range of movement, or stiffness, can all develop quite quickly. Everything possible needs to be done to prevent these problems. Associated reactions in the upper limb should also be addressed because these will have an effect on other activities such as gait.

Pain is often prevalent in the upper limb and may be reduced by proper management in the early stages particularly. This includes correct positioning, teaching specific exercises, encouraging the person to look after the arm, as well as passive mobilisations and stretches. There are various other techniques which may be used in the management of the upper limb, such as functional electrical stimulation, splints and positioning aids. Botulinum toxin can be helpful in some cases to control spasticity.

The trunk (the bit in the middle!) is sometimes forgotten, but is of vital importance as it provides a stable base for both the upper, lower limbs and head to work from. People are frequently left sitting in inappropriate chairs without correct support, thereby reinforcing abnormal patterns of movement and allowing the trunk to become weak and ineffective. A wheelchair can be a useful piece of equipment in the short/long term because it can provide a good sitting posture and may allow more freedom of movement.

The trunk may also have difficulty functioning correctly if the patient has been given a walking aid too early. By allowing someone to fix on to a stick or tripod, the whole dynamics of walking can alter. It is often very difficult to withdraw the aid at a late date when that person may feel unable to manage without it. High sticks can be useful for providing stability without compromising on posture. Simple activities such as rolling and unsupported sitting, may enable the trunk to become more mobile.

Lower limbs also require careful management and positioning in a similar way to the arm. It is particularly important to prevent tightness developing around the hip, knee and ankle. These can all affect the gait pattern quite markedly. Appropriate footwear is needed to provide correct support and stability. Some people may need more specialist advice with this, perhaps intervention from an orthotist, to help them to gain a stable base for weight bearing.

Bad habits or new problems can develop at any time. It is the role of neurological physiotherapists to analyse these changes. They can then help to develop a plan. This would integrate such treatment as is available locally with careful guidance to the patient. This would be aimed at high-lighting their role in their own recovery. A more positive outcome will always occur where there is appropriate support and explanation to stroke patients from those who are involved in their care.

CHAPTER 7

Functional Electrical Stimulation – the Odstock Dropped Foot Stimulator

PAUL TAYLOR AND JANE BURRIDGE

FUNCTIONAL ELECTRICAL STIMULATION (FES) was first used by the American bioengineer, W T Liberson, to help people who had had a stroke to lift their affected foot when walking. For some time after this the idea was not developed mainly because the technology was neither reliable nor user-friendly. The principle of FES is to replace the nerve impulses that are interrupted by damage to the brain or spinal cord with small electrical signals. It can be used not only with people who have had a stroke, but also people with spinal cord or head injuries, MS or cerebral palsy. It seems that it is particularly useful when people have spasticity – muscle stiffness.

Since Liberson's time there has been a considerable global research effort, the majority of which has been aimed at systems to help the spinal cord injured. However, more recently, attention has been turned towards stroke and some systems are beginning to become available. During the last fifteen years research at the Salisbury District Hospital has been attempting to make FES more effective and useful, by developing equipment and the clinical techniques and service. The people who are most likely to benefit are those who have a drop-foot, that causes them either to trip or hitch their hip when they walk. Work is also being done to apply the techniques to be useful with people who have some arm function but who, for example, lack the ability to open the hand even though they have quite a good grip.

Drop-foot

Drop-foot following stroke is a common problem. The condition prevents the patient from effectively swinging the leg when walking, causing an abnormal gait. The increased effort required not only means that walking is slow, tiring and sometimes unsafe, due to tripping, but may lead to further increase in spasticity.

Drop-foot is conventionally corrected by splinting, usually by a plastic ankle foot orthosis and, occasionally, a more substantial splint attached to the shoe. Many patients find the splint uncomfortable, sometimes exacerbating ankle oedema. In some cases patients do not find splinting an effective way of overcoming drop-foot, it may in fact lead to a further increase in calf tone and other problems.

The Odstock Dropped Foot Stimulator (ODFS) is a single-channel, foot-switch-triggered stimulator designed to elicit dorsiflexion of the foot by stimulation of the common peroneal nerve and is a direct development of a device first described by Liberson. The stimulator is about the size of a pack of cards and can be worn at the waist on a belt, or in a pocket. Leads connect the stimulator to the switch and the electrodes on the leg. Self-adhesive skin-surface electrodes are placed over the common peroneal nerve as it passes over the head of the fibula bone and the motor point, that is where the nerve enters the muscle, of tibialis anterior. The rise and fall of the stimulation can be adjusted to prevent a stretch reflex in the calf muscles, which is a significant component of spasticity. The device after a few days of practice, can be used all day as an orthotic aid or a training aid in gait re-education.

The ODFS was the subject of a randomised controlled trial (RCT)in which 32 stroke patients who had had a stroke for in excess of 6 months were allocated to a treatment group or a control group. The treatment group used the device and also received 12 sessions of physiotherapy, while the control group, who received the same contact time, only received physiotherapy. After three months of use the treatment group showed a statistically significant increase in walking speed and a reduction in the physiological cost index (PCI) when the stimulator was used, while no changes were seen in the control group. No significant 'carry-over' effect was seen, although a trend was present. Users of the ODFS showed a continuing reduction in quadriceps spasticity, which was only seen in the control group while physiotherapy continued. The treatment group also showed a reduction in the Hospital Anxiety and Depression index, suggesting an improvement in quality of life which was not seen in the control group. Of the 32 subjects at the start of the trial, 8 were using a splint, 13 had rejected this means of correction and 11 had either been advised not to use it or had not been offered it. All subjects in this trial who used electrical stimulation to correct drop-foot continued with this method in preference to conventional splinting.

The trial results were presented to the South and West Development and Evaluation Committee who, after examining this and evidence from other groups, subsequently recommended the ODFS for use in the UK's National Health Service.

Following the establishment of a clinical service, it was decided to continue recording the main outcome measures of walking speed and PCI that had been recorded in the RCT. An audit of these parameters over the first 18 weeks of use, confirmed the results of the original RCT and also showed a significant carry-over effect, i.e. an improvement in walking ability when not using the stimulator, in a group of 111 stroke subjects. A questionnaire survey indicated that the most common reasons for using the device were that it reduced the effort of walking, reduced tripping and improved confidence. Compliance was 92 per cent at 18 weeks and 86 per cent at one year. In the year 2000 the device was recommended by the Royal College of Physicians in their publication *National clinical guidelines on stroke*.

Other uses of the stimulators

While the ODFS is effective for many users, there often remains other gait problems. These can be addressed by stimulating additional muscle groups. A second device, the Odstock 2 Channel Stimulator, has been developed for this purpose. By stimulation of the hamstrings, knee flexion can be improved or the gluteus maximus muscle can be used to give hip extension while weight bearing. Other applications include bilateral dropped-foot and the stimulation of the triceps muscle to improve arm swing and, therefore, balance in gait. Another development, which is in the preliminary trial stages, is an implanted dropped-foot stimulator. Two different approaches are currently being investigated. The first, from Holland, uses a two channel implanted stimulator, one channel for each branch of the common peroneal nerve. In this way it is possible to independently control the amount of dorsiflexion (foot lift) and eversion (foot twisting outwards) allowing an accurate control of the foot's movements. Like the ODFS this device uses a foot switch. A second approach, this time from Denmark, uses a multichannel nerve cuff on the common peroneal nerve, which again allows selection of different movements. A novel feature of this system is that the researchers plan to pick up nerve signals from the sole of the foot to detect when the foot is placed on, or taken off, the floor. This has been shown to work in the laboratory but as yet is not available for home use.

Further research

Research is also being done to attempt to improve hand, arm and shoulder function. Shoulder subluxation is a common problem following stroke and is due to the in-ability of the shoulder muscles to maintain the humerus bone in its socket. This is often associated with pain. It has been shown that exercising using electrical stimulation, can reduce the subluxation and often eliminate shoulder pain. Similar exercises are also used for the hand and it has been shown that the voluntary range of movement can be improved and spasticity can be reduced. Anecdotally it has been claimed that these exercises can improve hand function, hastening recovery and it has also been suggested that sensory ability may also be improved.

Research is under way in several centres to produce a functional orthosis for the hand that would work in a similar way to the ODFS. At the time of writing, these devices have not entered regular clinical service, but promise useful benefit in the future. One approach is to use sensitive amplifiers to pick the residual electrical activity from the partially paralysed muscles and use this to control electrical stimulation, boosting the activity of the muscle. Other systems have suggested using other body-worn sensors to detect the user's intention to open their hand. As with drop-foot, implanted systems are also being considered.

It is likely that a useful device will become available over the next 10 years.

For more information about FES clinical service and research in Salisbury District Hospital with many links to other FES sites please check our web site: www.salisburyfes.com

References

1   Liberson W, Holmquest H, Scott M. 'Functional electrotherapy: stimulation of the common peroneal nerve synchronised with the swing phase of gait of hemiplegic subjects', *Archives of Physical Medicine and Rehabilitation*, 1961, 42, pp. 202–5.

2   Burridge J, Taylor P, Hagan S, Swain I. 'Experience of clinical use of the Odstock Dropped Foot Stimulator', *Artificial Organs*, 1997, 21(3), pp. 254–60.

3   Burridge J, Taylor P, Hagan S, Wood D, Swain I. 'The effects of common peroneal nerve stimulation on the effort and speed of walking: a randomised controlled clinical trial with chronic hemiplegic patients', *Clinical Rehabilitation*, 1997, 11, pp. 201–10.

4   Burridge J, Taylor P, Hagan S A, Wood D E, Swain I D. 'The effect on the spasticity of the quadriceps muscles of stimulation of the common peroneal nerve of chronic hemiplegic subjects during walking'. *Physiotherapy*, 1997, vol. 83, no 2.

5   Taylor P N, Burridge J H, Wood D E, Norton J, Dunkerly A, Singleton, C, Swain I D. 'Clinical use of the Odstock Drop Foot Stimulator – its effect on the speed and effort of walking', *Archives of Physical Medicine and Rehabilitation*, 1999, 80, pp. 1577–83.

6   Benson K and Hartz A J. 'A comparison of observational studies and randomized controlled trials', *N Engl J Med*, 2000, 342, pp. 1878–86.

7   Taylor P N, Burridge J H, Dunkerley A L, Lamb A, Wood D E, Norton J A, Swain I D. 'Patient's Perceptions of the Odstock Dropped Foot Stimulator (ODFS)', *Clinical Rehabilitation*, 1999, 13, pp. 333–40.

8   Intercollegiate working party for stroke. 'National clinical guidelines for stroke', 2000, London, Royal College of Physicians, (ISBN 1860 161 200).

9   Baker L L, Yeh C, Wilson D, Waters R L. 'Electrical stimulation of wrist and fingers for hemiplegic patients', Physical Therapy, 1979, 59 (12), pp. 1495–9.

10 Pandyan A D, Granat M H. 'Effects of electrical stimulation on flexion contractures in hemiplegics', Clinical Rehabilitation, 1997, 11, pp. 123–30.

11 Bowman B R, Baker L L, Waters R L. 'Position feedback and electrical stimulation: an automated treatment for hemiplegic wrist', Archives of Physical Medicines and Rehabilitation, Nov. 1979, Vol.60, pp. 497–501.

12 Kraft G H, Fitts S S and Hammond, M C. 'Techniques to improve function of the arm and hand in chronic hemiplegia', Archives of Physical Medicines and Rehabilitation, 1992, 73, pp. 220–7.

13 Prada G, Tallis R. 'Treatment of the neglect syndrome in stroke patients using a contingency stimulator', Clinical Rehabilitation, 1995, 9, pp. 304–13.

CHAPTER 8

The Bobath Concept*

MARGARET J MAYSTON

FOLLOWING THE RETIREMENT of Mrs Bobath from clinical practice and teaching in the late 1980s, there has been little or no literature by Bobath tutors to explain changes in philosophy or practice. The most commonly quoted reference to support Bobath as applied to the management of adults is the third and last edition of *Adult Hemiplegia* (Bobath, 1990) Similarly, for paediatrics the usually quoted work is Bobath and Bobath (1975).

According to these, the Bobath Concept uses the analysis of movement to determine what is necessary and possible for a client to achieve. The treatment ideas employed by the Bobaths were based on the knowledge available at the time, and assumed that spasticity was a problem of overactivity of the muscles resulting from abnormally enhanced tonic reflex activity. Accordingly it was thought that handling techniques inhibited such activity and made it possible for the person to achieve more normal movement.

Since then our understanding of the control of movement and spasticity has progressed. We know that tone, whether it is normal or abnormal, comprises both neural and non-neural components. Spasticity, classically referred to by Lance (1980) as a velocity-dependent increase in tonic stretch reflexes, is only one component of the movement dysfunction that may be encountered by people with neurological impairment, and in fact probably contributes very little to their movement disabilities.

* This section is based on 'Motor Learning Now Needs Meaningful Goals'. *Physiotherapy* September 2000/vol 86/no 9

Handling by itself cannot change spasticity (which represents the neural component of hypertonia), but may result in improved muscle length to allow for more efficient muscle activation. It is only by enabling the person to move more actively in more optimal and meaningful ways within the limits of their Central Nervous System damage that any reduction in the negative effects of spasticity can be achieved. While handling can be important in effecting changes in visco-elastic properties of muscle, activity is the key. It is not possible to effect normal activity in a CNS which has been significantly damaged, but the therapist can work with the client to optimise the remaining CNS tissue. The advances in neural plasticity, in particular the work of Nudo et al (see Nudo 1998 for a review) highlight the importance of activity to drive neuroplastic changes within the CNS. Therapists cannot directly inhibit spasticity (see Mayston 2002), but they can and must teach their clients to move in more efficient and functional ways.

Mrs Bobath at all times stressed the importance of activity, stating that although the handling was important, unless you make the person active you have 'done nothing at all'. (Bobath 1965). There is no good evidence to show that stopping a person from being active will prevent spasticity. This cannot be justified on scientific or financial grounds.

However, it should not be any activity. While it was thought that teaching people normal movement patterns and postural reactions would automatically lead to the performance of functional tasks, it is now known that the activity of the CNS is task dependent (Flament et al, 1993 and Ehrsson et al 2000). Therefore it is essential that therapists work with clients to achieve goals that are relevant to their lives, and not goals decided for them by therapists.

Bobath stressed the importance of common sense and

using 'what works'. Changes in both the understanding of the neurologically impaired person and the recognition that clinical presentations are often more complex than those clients on whom Mrs Bobath based her clinical observations and formulated her approach, also necessitates the need to modify clinical practice. The use of splints is not contra-indicated, but is seen as an adjunct to therapy, and can facilitate more efficient activity in other body parts. In addition, the use of pharmacological agents such as botulinum toxin, and other adjuncts such as functional electrical stimulation and muscle strengthening when used as a part of the process of achieving optimal functional ability of the person, can also be of value (Damiano and Abel 1998; Miller and Light, 1997)

Bobath-trained therapists are aware of the three main principles of motor learning:

1. Active participation

2. Opportunities for practice

3. Meaningful goals

The first two have always been important aspects of the application of the Bobath concept, but it is only in recent years that the importance of meaningful goals has been emphasised. Perhaps Bobath therapists have become so enthusiastic about changing tone that they have neglected the need to activate clients in meaningful ways.

Bobath trained therapists have excellent knowledge of the analysis of movement, a skill which can be complemented by current objective biomechanical and neuro-physiological measures of joint range, force output, reflex activity and muscle tone, in addition to the appropriate functional outcome measures. Therapists can then more effectively help clients achieve their optimal potential.

Where does this leave Bobath therapists? Is it time to recognise that we should acknowledge Mrs Bobath as a pioneer who was instrumental in changing clinical practice by recognising that every neurologically impaired person has a potential for improved activity in the affected body parts? Should we now go forwards, and not call what we do Bobath? Perhaps those who consider that they have taken the Bobath ideas forwards should consider putting their own names (or another name) to what they do and teach. Can we recognise the Bobath Centre as an important place to commemorate the contribution that Dr and Mrs Bobath made to neuro-rehabilitation, but realise that what is done within its walls attempts to encompass current knowledge and give clients their best possible chance to lead a better quality of life?

I speak as Director of the Bobath Centre when I state that we are not inhibiting abnormal reflexes, facilitating postural reactions and preventing clients from moving in ways which we think will increase their abnormal tone. Rather we work for optimal length and activity of muscles in a functional context, working with clients and families to determine what goals will improve the quality of life of all concerned. It is a process which requires ongoing self-education and evaluation.

References

Bobath B. 'Notes on Reflex Inhibiting Postures', *archival material*, Bobath Centre, London.

Bobath B. *Adult hemiplegia: Education and Treatment*, Heinemann Medical Books, 1990, Oxford, 3rd ed.

Bobath B and Bobath K. *Motor development in Different Types of Cerebral Palsy*, Heinemann Medical Books, Oxford, 1975.

Damiano D L and Abel L F. 'Functional Outcomes of Strength Training in Spastic Cerebral, Palsy. *Archives of Physical Medicine and Rehabilitation*, 1998, 79, 2, pp. 119–25

Ehrsson H H, Fagergren A, Jonsson T, Westling G, Johansson R and Forssberg H. 'Cortical activity in precision versus power grip tasks: an MRI study', *Journal of Neurophysiology*, 2000, 83, 1, pp. 528–36.

Flament D, Goldsmith P, Buckley J C, and Lemon R N. 'Task-dependence of EMG responses in first dorsal interosseous muscle to magnetic brain stimulation in man', *Journal of Physiology*, London, 2000, 464, pp. 361–72.

Lance J W. Symposium Synopsis. In 'Spasticity: Disordered Motor Control'. Editors: Feldman R G, Young R R, and Koella W O. *Chicago Year Book of Medical Publishers*, 1980, pages 485–95.

Mayston M J. 'Setting the scene' in: Edwards S (ed). *Neurological Physiotherapy: A problem solving approach*, Churchill Livingstone, Edinburgh, 2002, 2nd ed.

Miller G J T and Light K E. 'Strength training in spastic hemiparesis: Should it be avoided?', *Neurorehabilitation 9*, 1997, pp. 17–28.

Nudo R. 'Role of cortical plasticity in motor recovery after stroke', *Neurology Report*, 1998, 22, pp. 61–7.

CHAPTER 9

When words don't work – what to expect from speech and language therapy

DEBORAH HARDING

JUST TAKE A FEW MINUTES out to imagine yourself on a holiday overseas. It's a place where you do not speak the language very well but you are able to get by with a bit of rusty vocabulary you learnt at school and a phrase book. Unexpectedly you wake up in a hospital bed on a busy ward. You feel pretty groggy. There are tubes and charts all around. A nurse arrives, smiles and begins to talk to you. She speaks so fast. You think you caught a few words you recognised but can't quite remember what they mean. You think of things you want to ask – you've noticed your right arm and leg seem heavy and numb, you've got a headache, but how on earth do you understand what is going on? The few things you do manage to say are met with puzzled looks – your pronunciation's not up to much and after a few attempts your confidence is ebbing away and you're beginning to feel pretty anxious about speaking. It's scary and it's isolating and it resembles a little the experience of aphasia, the loss of language often associated with a left hemisphere stroke. Worse still for the person with aphasia, when family and friends turn up to visit they all seem to be speaking that strange, vaguely recognisable, language and they can't make any sense of what the patient is saying to them. (For fuller personal accounts see ref. 1.) At this point, hopefully, the friendly, smiling nurse reaches for the phone and makes a referral to the speech and language therapy department.

Communication and swallowing after a stroke

Aphasia, the loss of language, is just one of the communication impairments that can be part of the clinical picture following a stroke and occurs in about a third of all cases. Also encountered are voice problems: dysphonia, articulation problems; dysarthria and perhaps motor programming problems for speech, and dyspraxia. Co-existing with these communication problems and often the first reason an individual who has had a stroke meets a speech and language therapist – may be a swallowing problem, dysphagia. In addition there's an often overlooked area of communication problems associated with a right hemisphere stroke, e.g. problems understanding the more subtle complexities of communication such as inferred meaning. Where aphasia is the result of a stroke (i.e. not as a result of transient ischaemic attack, head injury, progressive neurological condition or infection such as encephalitis), the estimated incidence and prevalence for aphasia in a population of 100,000 is shown below (see refs. 2 & 3). As the prevalence figures are greater than the incidence of aphasia it goes without saying that many people who experience aphasia will require ongoing support and assistance, sometimes for years after the initial stroke.

Incidence	Prevalence		
per 100,000	per 100,000 of the population at any given time		
	moderate disability	severe/chronic disability	total
66	70	80	150

Services for people with aphasia

So, what support and services might be available if you experience communication or swallowing problems following a stroke? Whatever is written here will not reflect individual experience nor will it constitute a directory of services that will, should, or need to be provided. Each individual's needs will vary greatly. Additionally there is geographical variation in provision and there will be variation in individual clinicians: experience, creativity, area of special interest and philosophy. That said the Royal College of Speech and Language Therapists has been proactive in the introduction of professional standards and clinical guidelines to ensure best practice throughout the profession. Speech and language therapists working in the National Health Service are required to be registered members of the Royal College of Speech and Language Therapists. To re-register each year the therapist is required to complete a certain amount of continuing professional development, a written record of which must be witnessed by a fellow member. Perhaps most reassuring is that the field of aphasiology is an area rich with both clinical and academic researchers, employing both quantitative and qualitative methodologies to evaluate therapeutic interventions. Treatment efficacy has been widely demonstrated in specific impairments: the ability to communicate in everyday situations and, more broadly, in terms of social, emotional and psychological well-being.

The increased involvement seen in the 1980s and 1990s of the speech and language therapy profession in the assessment and management of swallowing problems put a strain on departmental resources. Many in the profession feared that the 'quality of life' communication work became a less pressing priority than the 'life and death' of swallowing problems. In an acute hospital environment speech and language therapists contribute much to improving the quality of people's lives following strokes by assessing and treating swallowing disorders. Such expertise will certainly have saved many from the misery and risks of aspiration pneumonia.

In hospitals where there is an established speech and language therapy department ward staff will know how to get the therapist along to see someone in their care. Even so it is worth knowing that speech and language therapy operates an open referral system, i.e. anyone can make a referral – professional, relative or the individual seeking assistance. The only exception to this will be where a swallowing assessment is required. The potential impact on medical condition of assessment and intervention for swallowing necessitates a doctor's referral. Bedside assessment is often the first contact and will involve, though not necessarily all in one go, a screening of communication problems, advice to facilitate communication on the ward, an invitation to family/next of kin to contact the speech and language therapist if they were not seen on the ward, information about communication problems and other useful organisations, e.g. Speakability, Connect, The Stroke Association or Headway, (see useful organisations on page 96). The advice at this stage can seem like a lot of common sense, coupled with a fair amount of reluctance (from the therapist) to respond definitively to questions about longer term outcome and ultimate recovery of speech. It's easy to forget just how complicated the human language is! In speaking, words come and go in fractions of seconds. For the normal listener, with language processing intact, each snippet of sound is speedily processed and a system of prediction about what will come next or what is required next will be operating, based on the listener's sophisticated knowledge of normal language. The following illustration is striking in speech but it works reasonably in writing too: If you hear someone say 'She used the knife to. . . . .' the listener just can't help a word popping into her head to fill the gap, e.g. cut or spread, etc. In contrast consider this example: Her husband rolled in drunk again and in a fit of rage she used the knife to . . .' and a different word may spring to mind. If a normal language user can be this sophisticated at such a small scale the language patterns observed in aphasia seem a little less mysterious. It becomes possible to imagine that there need only be a minor hiccup in language processing to derail the system spectacularly and, of course, following a stroke there's very likely been a more major derailment.

What happens beyond the acute hospital varies from service to service. It may include regular therapy, review, an invitation to contact the department if problems persist or an out-patient appointment on discharge from the hospital. For some, once medically stable, there may be a period of further in-patient rehabilitation at a specialist stroke or neuro-rehabilitation unit. In general this occurs where the individual is experiencing more extensive or complex physical, cognitive and communication disability, requiring multidisciplinary management.

Theoretical influences on therapy approaches

Aphasiology is an area rich with the highest level of clinical and academic interest. The multidisciplinary membership of organisations such as the British Aphasiology Society, (see useful organisations on page 96), are evidence of this. As a result aphasia therapy is underpinned by extensive research and founded in recognised and developed theories of language processing and communicative behaviour.

WHO classifications

Like all rehabilitation professionals the speech and language therapist will be mindful of the World Health Organisation classifications of Impairment, Activity and Participation (see ref 4). Do these classifications matter in speech and language therapy intervention and what do they mean? A good illustration in communication terms would be where the impairment was one of inability to spell exceptional words, i.e. those that do not conform to normal spelling rules. The impact on activity might be that the person's writing is littered with regularised spelling mistakes and might be equivalent for people with similar levels of impairment. However the effect on a given individual's participation will vary according to the individual's need to be able to spell such words accurately. For example, the impact on participation for persons who make their living as proof readers will be much greater than the impact for persons who work as waiters. The table on page 91 illustrates this further.

Approaches to assessment and subsequent interventions initiated by speech and language therapists have developed and continue to develop, in these three areas.

Addressing impairments

Impairment level approaches underwent major revision in the 1980s and 1990s as cognitive neuro-psychological theories of language processing and breakdown began to influence clinicians. A more problem-solving approach to communication problems following a stroke or other brain injury developed and, together with other theoretically motivated approaches addressing the impairment level there is now substantial evidence to suggest that aphasia therapy is efficacious, (see refs. 5, 6, & 7). Furthermore, specific clinical assessment tools have been developed to assess impairment (see refs. 8 & 9). The impairment level approaches are sometimes accused of having little functional relevance, i.e. little to offer at an activity or participative level. However, the theoretically driven impairment approaches do enable therapists to apply 'hosepipe theory' to aphasia, i.e. if there's no water coming out of the hose it could be for any number of reasons – the tap is not on, there's a perforation in the hose, there's a kink in the hose, the water supply has been cut off, etc. Every cause produces the same effect but requires a different approach to resolve. Similarly, using a cognitive neuro-psychological perspective to illustrate, the inability to name an object can be the result of a breakdown at differing language processing levels such as word meanings (semantics), word sounds (phonology), short term storage or articulation. As for the view that impairment therapies do not address the functional impact of the language disorder for the individual, creative clinicians strive to make even the simplest semantic (word meaning) therapy task functionally relevant by, for example, using words or other stimuli that have functional relevance to a given individual. In so doing the clinician will also counter concern about item-specific improvement or carry-over to non-treated items. Furthermore, theoretical models of language processing can serve to provide some order and rationale for the chaotic speech, writing or comprehension patterns that form the surface and lay perception of aphasia. Interestingly, models of language processing are now an integral part of research into the functional neuro-anatomy of communication, i.e. which bits of the brain do the processing necessary for communication (see ref. 10) and are being computer-tested both as models of normal function and to explore whether, when lesioned, these

Problems (impairments)	Impact of problems on daily life (activity/participation)
Difficulty understanding simple spoken sentences	Cannot follow conversations Often chooses the wrong drink when offered a selection Only follows simple one-to-one conversation Cannot enjoy television/radio
Word finding problem	Limited participation in conversation Difficulty telling people how she/he is feeling Relies on partner to finish sentences Unable to use telephone effectively
Difficulty spelling exception/irregular words	Slower writing letters College assignments have increased spelling errors Unable to keep up with note keeping in meetings/lectures
Poor self-monitoring	Doesn't notice when the words she/he produces are mispronounced Doesn't notice when she/he says the wrong word Is unaware she/he has difficulty understanding Doesn't recognise listeners' difficulty understanding him/her
Reading comprehension poor for complex syntactic structures	Unable to follow recipes Misunderstands official correspondence Requires assistance to manage personal correspondence

theoretical models produce impaired performance analogous to aphasic patterns (see ref. 11). What is not conclusively known, as yet, is whether there is a critical time for aphasia therapy to be effective. There is some suggestion that therapeutic intervention needs to be reasonably intensive, perhaps five hours per week. While assessment and the development and evaluation of therapeutic programmes would require a trained therapist, the daily practice could take the form of independent work or work with an appropriately briefed professional or lay person such as a healthcare assistant, volunteer or family member. Of course, professionals and loved ones need to be mindful that, while for some such roles can be a positive and empowering experience, for others it can be a tense, negative and destructive activity.

Looking beyond impairment

Speech and language therapy for aphasia is not solely about restoration of linguistic or cognitive function. At an early stage there should be some consideration of facilitating the individual's immediate communication needs. It cannot be assumed, although professionals and families often do, that the person with aphasia will be able to write or read instead of speaking. Perhaps even more surprising is that a person experiencing aphasia may not be able to use gesture to communicate either. Even those individuals with the physical, motor ability to make gestures may need encouragement and facilitation to recognise that such gestural skills can be used communicatively. It does not follow that a person with some understanding of single written words will be able to point to written words to convey messages or use a sophisticated, technologically advanced communication aid (see ref. 12). Conversely, assessment may reveal some intact processing which may be employed almost un-facilitated as an effective compensatory strategy (see ref. 13). So aphasia can involve the breakdown of the diverse aspects of symbolism and processing that form human communication in unexpected and surprising ways. Skilled speech and language therapy assessment will identify processes which may be employed successfully to facilitate communication. At this point the two-way nature of communication needs to be acknowledged and within the field of aphasia therapy there is increasing work encouraging the development and training of conversation partners for people with communication problems (see ref. 14), perhaps in tandem with specific linguistic therapy.

Psychosocial and emotional well-being

Inevitably there is a psychosocial and emotional impact of aphasia for the individual and those around him/her. The need to acknowledge, explore and provide support in this respect has always been recognised by the speech and language therapy profession. Furthermore, at Connect, for example, a counselling service is offered by trained counsellors with personal experience of aphasia

Living with aphasia

Earlier in this chapter the more enduring nature of aphasia was eluded to in considering the prevalence figures. Perhaps, because speech and language therapy has developed predominately within a medicine-led health service, the longer term needs have received less attention until recently. Hard-pressed health resources have focused on timely discharge. The speech and language therapy profession has always brought wide ranging skills to the support of all people with communication problems and openly and actively

93

included families and carers in rehabilitation programmes. The long term impact of aphasia for individuals and those around them is now becoming a central area of the interest for clinical and research aphasiologists alike, (see ref. 15). Research in this domain embraces social models of disability and qualitative research methodologies, such as ethnography. These extensive and varied approaches generally look beyond the linguistic though some, such as the training of conversation partners, represent a marriage of applied clinical linguistics and social facilitation (see ref. 16). Importantly there has been a move to develop aphasia-friendly resources (see ref. 17) and to include people with aphasia in the planning and development of services.

In summary, aphasia is as varied as it is complex. The assessment and treatment require methodical, creative, inclusive and empathetic approaches ranging from common sense advice to complex psycholinguistic programmes of therapy. Encouragingly, the wealth of published research in aphasiology suggests speech and language therapy is effective and professional support for the person with aphasia should always form part of the multidisciplinary network required for the effective delivery of a service to the survivors of strokes.

References

1   Parr S, Byng S, Gilpin S and Ireland C. *Talking about Aphasia: Living with Language Loss after Stroke*, OUP, 1997.

2   Enderby P and Phillip R. 'Speech and Language Handicap: Towards knowing the size of the problem',*British Journal of Disorders of Communication*, 1986, 21 (2), pp. 151–65.

3   Enderby P and Davies P. 'Communication disorders: Planning a service to meet the needs', *British Journal of Disorders of Communication*, 1989, 24, pp. 301–31.

4   WHO-Disability Functioning ICIDH-2 International classification of impairments, activities and participation

5   Byng S. 'Hypothesis Testing and Aphasia Therapy', in Holland A and Forbes M (Eds), *Aphasia Treatment – World Perspectives*, 1993, San Diego: Singular, pp. 115–30.

6   Harding D and Pound C. 'Needs, Function and Measurement: Juggling with multiple language impairment', in Byng S, Swinburn K and Pound C, (Eds), *The Aphasia Therapy File*, Hove: Psychology Press, 1999.

7   Nickels L and Best W. 'Therapy for naming disorders (Part I): principles, puzzles and progress'. *Aphasiology*, 1996, 10 (1), pp. 21–47.

    Nickels L and Best W. 'Therapy for naming disorders (Part I): specifics, surprises and suggestions', *Aphasiology*, 1996, 10 (2), pp. 109–36

8   Kay J, Lesser R, and Coltheart M. *Psycholoinguistic assessments of language processing in aphasia*. Hove, UK: Psychology Press, 1992.

9   Whitworth A, Perkins L, and Lesser R. *Conversation analysis profile for people with aphasia*. London: Whurr, 1997.

10 Wise R J S, Scott S K, Blank S C, Mummery C J, Murphy K, and Warburton E A. 'Separate Neural Sub-systems within "Wernicke's Area"', *Brain*, 2001, 124, pp. 83–95.

11 Martin N and Saffran E M. 'A computational account of deep dysphasia', *Brain and Language*, 1992, 43, pp. 240–274.

12 Harding D and Pound C. 'Needs, Function and Measurement: Juggling with multiple language impairment'. In Byng S, Swinburn K and Pound C, (Eds), *The Aphasia Therapy File*, Hove: Psychology Press, 1999.

13 Howard D and Harding D. 'Self-cueing of word retrieval by a woman with aphasia : why a letter board works', *Aphasiology*, 1998, 12 (4/5), pp. 399–420.

14 Kagan A. 'Supported conversation for adults with aphasia: methods and resources for training conversation partners', *Aphasiology*, 1998,12 (9), pp. 816–830.

15 Pound C, Parr S, Lindsay J and Woolf C. 'Beyond Aphasia', *Therapies for Living with Communication Disability*, London: Winslow, 2000.

16 Lock S, Wilkinson R and Bryan K. 'Supporting Partners of People with Aphasia'. In *Relationships and Conversations* (SPPARC), London: Winslow 2001.

17 Parr S, Pound C, Byng S and Long B. *The Aphasia Handbook*, Ecodistribution, Leicestershire, 1999.

Useful organisations

CONNECT

The communication disability network
16–18 Marshalsea Street
London SE1 1HL
Tel: 020 7367 0840

THE STROKE ASSOCIATION

Stroke House, Whitecross Street
London EC1Y 8JJ
Tel: 020 7490 7999

SPEAKABILITY

1 Royal Street, London SE1 7LL
Tel: 020 7261 9572

HEADWAY

National Head Injuries Association
4 King Edward Court, King Edward Street
Nottingham NG1 1EW
Tel: 0115 924 0800

THE BRITISH APHASIOLOGY SOCIETY   www.bas.org.uk

CHAPTER 10

Cognitive problems following stroke

KIT MALIA **and** ANNE BRANNAGAN

THE MAJORITY OF PEOPLE who suffer a stroke will notice they have changed in a number of ways; the most obvious of these are the physical and speech difficulties. However, many people will also notice problems with their cognitive skills.

What is cognition?

Basically cognition is defined as anything to do with thinking and learning. Our cognitive skills allow us to make sense of the world around us as well as our inner world (our feelings and thoughts). There are many different components that go to make up cognition. These can be divided into five main areas: attention, visual processing, information processing, memory and executive functions.

Attention

This is the foundation of all other cognitive skills. Without good control of our attention we will definitely have difficulties with all other aspects of our cognition. You may experience these difficulties if you have attention problems:

Difficulties concentrating
Difficulties with ignoring background distractions
Difficulties in picking out the most important thing on
    which to attend at any given time

Difficulties in moving your attention fluidly between
different ideas or tasks

Difficulty in doing more than one thing at the same time.

Visual processing

This includes our ability to move our eyes, to focus on
things, to match patterns, visual fields (the amount we can
see around us without moving our heads), as well as visual
perception (making sense of the visual information). If you
have problems with visual processing you may experience
the following difficulties in your everyday life:

Bumping into furniture, doors or people

Difficulty with reading

Difficulty watching TV

Double vision

Blurred vision.

Information processing

This is a general term that covers most aspects of cognition
as defined above. However, after stroke there appear to be
three major aspects that require rehabilitation: speed of
thinking, capacity of thinking, and control of the organisation processes. If you have any of the following problems
they may indicate difficulties with information processing:

Finding you get lost in conversations with more than
one person

Finding you cannot think of things to say, particularly
when in busy environments

Feeling that you think more slowly or less clearly

Finding that you seem to 'get hold of the wrong end of
the stick' a lot of the time

Memory

This is the cognitive skill that most people complain about. However, problems with memory are often due to difficulties with attention or information processing skills. By successfully working on, and improving, these areas memory complaints may then subside. The most disabling aspects of memory failures are:

Difficulty remembering things that have happened recently (episodic memory)

Difficulty remembering to do things in the future e.g. keeping appointments, what to buy at the shop etc (prospective memory)

Executive functions

These can be likened to the conductor of the orchestra; they co-ordinate all the other cognitive functions. If there are problems with executive functions then problems can occur with any aspect of cognition. Problems in this area tend to be more subtle to define, although the effects of them are very disabling. You may experience any of the following:

Difficulties with planning
Difficulties with setting appropriate goals
Difficulties with self-monitoring
Difficulties with awareness
Difficulties with getting started on things

How do I know if I have cognitive problems?

You could arrange assessment via a clinical or neuro-psychologist in order to formally document your problems and their severity. However, if you are unable to do this then by simply talking with relatives and friends about the potential problems as listed above, you should gain a better idea of the extent of your difficulties. It is likely that most people will have at least some self-awareness of their own cognitive changes.

Treatment approaches

Cognitive Rehabilitation Therapy aims to maximise or optimise cognitive skills. There are four approaches which need to be included, although the relative amount of each component will vary from individual to individual:

- **Education** – it is essential that the individual knows what their difficulties are, what has caused them, in what circumstances they tend to be most apparent, and what they can do about them. Without good education then self-awareness cannot develop. Awareness is the key to successful rehabilitation. The better the awareness, the more likely the individual will be able to benefit from cognitive rehabilitation.

- **Process training** – this involves completing exercises that have been designed to target specific cognitive difficulties. They are usually pen and paper or computer-based tasks. They do not have direct relevance to everyday life tasks, but rather focus on the underlying skills which enable us to perform these tasks. This kind of training is very useful as an educational tool and for strategy training as well, since the tasks are easy to quantify, usually relatively quick to complete, can be repeated many times, and can be graded in increasing amounts of difficulty. They also appear to have a marked effect on improving confidence and self-esteem. The aim behind process training is to improve the actual brain function.

- **Strategy training** – the aim behind strategy training is to provide a method of minimising the effect of the cognitive problem through application of a technique or strategy. The problem is still there, but the strategy stops it being a problem. External and internal strategies can be used. The former are things that can be seen, touched, heard etc, whereas the former are things that are done inside your own head. It is generally better to focus on developing the use of external strategies, such as list writing, calendars, notes, visual prompts, diaries, electronic alarms etc.

- **Functional activities training** – it is absolutely essential to apply what is learned via the education, process training and strategy training, into real life activities. Without this aspect the others become relatively meaningless. On the other hand just doing functional activities is too general and does not allow the same level of analysis of what is causing the failures, and tends to lead to problems with generalisation of skills to novel situations in everyday life. All four aspects need to be used together for maximum effect.

Resources for cognitive rehabilitation

Education

Distance Learning Course in Cognitive Rehabilitation.
(Available from www.braintreetraining.co.uk)

The Nature of Memory, CD Rom
(Available from www.memoryzine.com)

Head Injury: A Practical Guide (1994) – T Powell – and a range of other useful publications.
(Available from www.headway.org.uk)

Introduction to Cognitive Rehabilitation: Theory and Practice (1989).
Sohlberg M M & Mateer C A. The Guilford Press,
New York.

Cognitive Rehabilitation: An integrative Neuro-psychological Approach
(2001). Sohlberg M M & Mateer C A. The Guilford Press,
New York.

Caring for Carers: Cognitive Functions Workshop. Malia & Brannagan.
(Available from www.braintreetraining.co.uk)

Process training

Brainwave-R: Cognitive Strategies and Techniques for Brain Injury
Rehabilitation. (Available in Europe from Brain Tree
Training, PO Box 79, Leatherhead, Surrey, KT23 4YT,
UK – www.braintreetraining.co.uk Available in USA
from ProEd, 8700 Shoal Creek Boulevard, Austin, Texas
78757-6897, USA – www.proedinc.com)

Attention Process Training (Parts 1 and 2). (Available from Lash
& Associates Publishing/Training Inc, 708 Young Forest
Drive, Wake Forest, North Carolina 27587-9040, USA –
www.lapublishing.com

Ideas from educational materials and puzzle books, readily
available from a browse in a suitable bookshop.

Neurotraining materials (general stimulation ideas) (Craine
J F & Gudeman H E (1981). The Rehabilitation of Brain
Functions. Charles C Thomas Publishers, Springfield, IL.)

Various computer-based exercise programmes, including
the following: Cognitive rehabilitation series (available
from Hartley Courseware Inc, 123 Bridge Rd, Box 419,
Dimondale, MI 48821, USA); Psychological Software
services – a range of software (available from PSS Inc,

6555 Carrollton Avenue, Indianapolis, IN 46220, USA);
The NeurXercise System, (available from NeurX
Corporation, 10905 Fort Washington Rd, Suite 108,
Fort Washington, MD 20744, USA); Captains Log
(available from 727 Twin Ridge Lane, Richmond, VA
23235, USA). There are many more computer-based
programmes available which can be located relatively
easily via searches on the internet.

Cognitive Rehabilitation Workbook (In press). Powell T & Malia K B

How to do Cognitive Rehabilitation (In press).
Malia K B & Brannagan A E.

Strategies
How to do Cognitive Rehabilitation (In Press).
Malia K B & Brannagan A E.

Caring for Carers: Cognitive Functions Workshop.
Malia K B & Brannagan A E.
(Available from www.braintreetraining.co.uk)

Cognitive Rehabilitation of Memory: A practical guide. (1992).
Harrell M, Parente F, Bellingrath E G & Lisicia K A Aspen
Publishers, Gaithersburg M A, USA.

Functional activities
Basically any activity that forms a part of the individual's
normal day can be used, e.g. television, sports, shopping,
cooking, etc. What makes these activities part of the cognitive rehabilitation programme is the way in which they
are structured. Just watching television is not a cognitive
therapeutic activity – it is leisure; but providing a worksheet
with specific things to look out for and report on would
make a sports programme or a soap opera programme a

cognitive therapeutic activity. For more ideas on this see the following:

Caring for Carers: Cognitive Functions Workshop.
Malia K B & Brannagan A E.
(Available from www.braintreetraining.co.uk)

How to do Cognitive Rehabilitation (In Press).
Malia K B & Brannagan A E.

Distance Learning Course in Cognitive Rehabilitation.
(Available from www.braintreetraining.co.uk)

Additional useful websites

www.nanonline.org – website for the National Academy of Neuro-psychology, USA
www.cognitive-rehab.org.uk – website for the Society for Cognitive Rehabilitation

CHAPTER 11

Different doctors –
a personal view*

PROFESSOR D L MCLELLAN

DOCTORS TEND TO BE CRITICISED for focusing too much on diseases and not enough on the people who have them. Someone who experiences a stroke needs to be able to explore with their doctor not only what a stroke is, but how to understand and cope with the experience, and then how best to face the future. This means that doctors need to understand not only the medical aspects of stroke, but equally the turmoil experienced by the patient and family and the processes by which this turmoil can be worked through during rehabilitation.

This is a tall order for doctors and especially for young ones, most of whom have yet to experience in their own lives the upheaval of major life events. Many stroke patients have already experienced such life events and will certainly be experiencing one after their stroke. Yet it is junior hospital doctors who will be the first to see someone admitted to hospital after a stroke, and who will be the doctors most closely involved in their day-to-day experience when in hospital.

How do young doctors learn about the significance of stroke for a person's life story and sense of identity, without having to reach the same age and to have had the same experience as their patients? This is achieved partly through their formal education and training and crucially by the

* This article was first published in *Different Strokes*

example of their 'role models', their consultants. If their consultants are seen to give priority to understanding what the stroke means to their patients and what their fears are, then junior doctors will seek to do the same and will value this expertise in themselves. If, however, the consultant appears to be interested only in the diagnostic aspects of the stroke, and the use of drugs to treat it, and if the main expectation placed on the junior doctor is simply to get the patient discharged from hospital as soon as humanly possible, then this inadequate agenda will tend to be passed on to the next generation of consultants and so the cycle will be repeated.

Understanding the experience of stroke, and recognising the need to provide better help, is one of the major aims of the speciality of rehabilitation medicine. Britain's newest speciality, it was formally established across the UK for the first time only in 1989. From a base of about 15 consultants and 4 trainees in 1989 it has developed to over 120 consultants and 45 trainees today, and these numbers are expanding as fast as young doctors can be attracted into the speciality. What is different about rehabilitation? Most NHS rehabilitation services are organised with older, retired people in mind. However, younger people have different agendas in their rehabilitation. Disabled school leavers may be seeking to establish themselves independently as young adults for the first time. A little later they will be grappling with the early stages of their adult careers, where the increasing demands of work and family will create different priorities. More intensive therapies and demanding treatments will be appropriate for younger people with greater physical energy, whose lives are still being carved out.

Young doctors training in rehabilitation medicine are taught the importance of understanding the meaning of stroke to younger individuals and families who experience one. They are taught that, while two strokes may appear much the same, two people with strokes never are and that the attributes and objectives of the person who has a stroke are crucial elements in negotiating what rehabilitation should aim at and what form it should take. To serve younger people in the UK effectively we need at least 250 consultants. We currently have 110. We need to get an equally strong commitment from social services, local councils, the voluntary sector and the employment and education services.

One of the challenges in rehabilitation generally is to promote areas of knowledge and the specific practices of each profession, at the same time as ensuring that they work together as members of a genuine rehabilitation team when they need to. When professions are young they tend to be unsure of their role and status and they are instinctively better at competing than at collaborating across boundaries. However, in the past 15 years there has been a transformation of the academic base of the therapy professions, who are now established in universities and who have increasingly adopted the university tradition of multi-disciplinary and inter-disciplinary research and training. Britain developed the world's first national multidisciplinary research society, the Society for Research into Rehabilitation, which rapidly grew into a thriving scientific body, with international links across the world. At Society of Rehabilitation meetings (the proceedings of which are regularly published in the scientific journal *Clinical Rehabilitation*), new research can be debated in a multi-professional setting.

Sounds very grand, doesn't it? But when will I see results (I hear you ask) in the behaviour of doctors in my local hospital, health centre or community NHS services? The answer is that you should be starting to see it already, especially if you have seen a consultant in rehabilitation medicine locally, or your doctor has been exposed to rehabilitation medicine during training. Our specialists are committed to working as closely as possible with the other rehabilitation professionals, and also with social and voluntary sector services. With them we are campaigning for unified management structures and budgets, and unified planning of development of services at each locality, in order to promote rehabilitation. Central to any such development is consumer involvement both in the planning and implementation of services. Organisations such as Different Strokes are very important players here.

The British Society of Rehabilitation Medicine is committed not only to improving specialist medical practice in rehabilitation, but to developing a fundamental concept in medical thinking and behaviour. Those shameful days when consultants on their 'rounds' would walk past stroke patients without even speaking to them should be a thing of the past but we recognise there is still a long way to go.

Part 3

STROKE AND DIFFERENT
AGE GROUPS:
CHILDREN, YOUNG ADULTS
AND THE ELDERLY

CHAPTER 12

Different age groups

T HE PUBLIC PERCEPTION of stroke is still that it only affects the elderly, but strokes can strike at any time of life. When it occurs to a young person or a child, the shock and disbelief is enormous. Information is hard to find, families feel isolated and, worse still, treatment and after care are often woefully inadequate or inappropriate.

Strokes and children

'Childhood stroke has been known for centuries. It is defined as any child between one month and sixteen years of age who has had a stroke. As in adults, there are many causes. Unlike adults, the number of children having strokes is unknown, but for the United Kingdom it is felt to be between 250 to 1000 cases per annum.'

This statement comes from the synopsis of the *National Childhood Stroke Study* (Dr A N Williams 1999) see page 155. The statistics may come as a surprise to parents faced with their child who has had a stroke. To them it is a singular experience and they will feel bewildered. It is likely that they will have not heard of a previous case and will be desperate for information about how to proceed after the acute stage is over.

Priorities are very different for the three age groups. Leaving aside the medical aspects, children need to be able to get back to school and continue their education as soon as possible. They need their friends as well as the under-standing of their teachers and education authorities for whatever support and assistance they may need. The time scale is so different. If a recovery, allowing an individual to take part in normal activities, takes a year or even two for someone much older, this might not be too serious – for a child this is a considerable period in their development. In education any period, once missed is hard to replace; even missing a term puts added strain as a pupil tries to catch up.

All ages of stroke patients tend to be left with some similar problems, but they may affect their daily life in slightly different ways. Take fatigue; it affects both performance and memory. A child may be competent at the beginning of the day – or week – and hardly remember a thing at the end. Will teachers understand? How accurate is an assessment taken at one extreme or another? Someone may appear to be competent when moving slowly and purposefully, but what happens when hurried? It is difficult to explain the upset that may occur when you are forced to try to perform any action at speed. Something like a fire practice at school, might induce real panic in a child. Particular worries are involved when changing from primary to secondary school. Will there be stairs without rails on both sides or even steps with no supports occasionally at the new site? Children hate to stand out as different – what will other children say? It is distressing to learn from parents how much some children worry about such things, even to the extent of not being able to sleep. Such tensions will affect all aspects of performance. There are common-sense solutions to many of these problems but how often are they dealt with in a sensitive way in an overstretched education system?

Echoing what Jane Cast said about adult patients needing help long after support had ceased (see page 65): child patients grow into adolescents with all the insecurities and problems involved. An emotional backlash would not be surprising as teenagers realise the implications of their condition. It would make little difference at that moment whether their worst fears were realistic or not, and a teenager might not be able or willing to voice them.

I would like to point out that what I have said on page 14 about handwriting, and what I recommend for adults may not necessarily be right for children. They need to be able to produce written work as soon as possible to keep up with their school work. Some children can adjust to using their non-preferred hand quite easily. One primary pupil I know developed an efficient writing quickly and found little difficulty in keeping up with his peers. Other children have lost the use of their non-preferred hand and so can still write, but there is a downside. In both circumstances I have noticed that the affected hand is not being used sufficiently (whether receiving therapy or not) to regain strength and usage without that motivation that the desire to write provides. The more the affected hand and arm are ignored the more one-sided the child will become (see pages 15 and 69).

One parent distinctly remembers a doctor saying that she should 'write off' her child's preferred hand as useless and concentrate on retraining the non-preferred one. By the time this was achieved and the implications realised she reported that it was too late, too tiring and dispiriting to do much about the situation. Everyone needs two efficient hands if possible, so a balanced attitude is desirable towards encouraging gradual and appropriate use of the preferred hand, but admittedly that balance is not easy to achieve.

An American friend sent me this apt quote that she found on an OT website: 'I have a four-year-old girl on my case-load who has right-side post-stroke involvement. One day she just came out and told me her hand doesn't work. I told her she's got to tell it to work better or it won't know. Well, she started saying to her hand, "Hand, work better!" and it did.' What an excellent way of explaining to a young child just what we adults usually have to find out for ourselves. Older patients should learn from this simple statement, because, believe me, telling your hand or foot what to do is exactly what you may need to do for quite some while before it learns to perform a certain action by itself.

My correspondent conjectured whether small children were better at 'mind over matter' than older people. It is that clear explanation that works whatever the age and it is wrong to suppose that young children are any less moti-vated to help themselves than someone older, once they are pointed in the right direction. There is another factor to consider. Child patients are not unintelligent and should be listened to, just like adults. Therapists are not invariably right. For instance, when prescribing aids – children may be able to feel what suits their body or meets their needs and what does not. Anyhow they are unlikely to make full use of something when they are not comfortable with it.

As a family, we learned a lot when our youngest daughter, then aged six, suffered a sudden, serious neurological condition not dissimilar to a stroke. Something like this affects the whole family. Parent's lives are obviously dis-rupted as they have to alter priorities, but what about siblings? They also suffer as their activities may be severely curtailed. Their own feelings can vary from acute distress to the perhaps more natural angry reaction for a young child of: 'Why should this happen to us. It's not fair'. It may be difficult for them to understand, however hard parents may try, why most of the focus must now be on the patient and his or her needs. This may have to be the case for many months, even years, creating real hardship. On the other hand it can unite everyone and strengthen family ties.

Attitudes of those around them affect young patients too. I wonder now how my own worries added to my daughter's so I asked her, 25 years later, what she remembered. She recalled that she was hypersensitive to hushed tones and funny looks. She was able to see through what she called doctors' and nurses' false cheerfulness and could tell when things were going wrong. 'Children tune in to body language', she says.

I will never forget the consultant who voiced a dire prognosis in front of my child. She revealed, by occasional comments, how well she had understood and how it preyed on her mind for several years before it became obvious that what was prophesied was not going to happen. We survived the first difficult year because we had the help of a wise paediatrician locally (the late Dr Peter Swift). There are, however, many positive factors to give parents hope. Children who go through such experiences become exceptionally motivated teenagers and sensitive, caring adults. They frequently overcome their difficulties in the end and delight in proving the experts wrong.

Across the country many parents of children recovering from a stroke feel isolated. They tell me that they deplore the lack of a network and helpline for parents. They stress the need for user-friendly leaflets (in different languages), preferably written by parents who have experience. They plead for a support group like Different Strokes, specially for parents of young child patients.

Dr Fenella Kirkham is a paediatric neurologist based at the Institute of Child Health and at Southampton General Hospital. She has a special interest in child stroke patients and has contributed a chapter, from the perspective of a consultant, outlining the possible causes, necessary investigations and likely treatments for a child with a stroke. She emphasises how families can help their own children, all of which is particularly valuable as the subject is so little understood. To have access to such information is important for all concerned with the care and guidance of children

Young adults

Each year over 10,000 people of working age in the UK have a stroke. Over 1000 of them are under the age of 30, reports the organisation Different Strokes. The following quotation comes from a summary of *A Study to Evaluate the Met and Unmet Needs of Young Stroke Survivors*, by D L McLellan, P Kersten, A Ashburn and A George (see also page 155):

'Although stroke is the most common cause of adult disability in the UK there is a lack of knowledge about an individual's perception of their own recovery. There is evidence to show that organised services for people with stroke can help to increase independence. There are also some indications that the needs of people who have had a stroke, and their carers are inadequately met.'

Many young stroke survivors would, I am sure, echo the last sentence. For young adults the main concern might be how they will be able to get back to work or their studies and support themselves and their families, as well as to live a full life in other ways. Being aware of the implications, and devastating affect on them and all around them, and yet with their whole lives before them, young stroke survivors deserve the very best treatment – but are they getting it? They have a champion in Donal O'Kelly. He was a barrister of twenty years, specialising in criminal and family law, who suffered a severe, brain stem stroke when in court. Because of the inadequacy in the system that he and other fellow stroke sufferers experienced he founded Different

Strokes to cater for the needs of young adults and those up to the age of fifty-five.

The annual conference of this organisation in 2000 gave a good idea of its various functions. First, there was a presentation on cognitive rehabilitation, by Kit Malia. He defined cognition as: 'The working of the mind through which we make sense of the world'. He analysed the various components under five headings: attention, visual processing, information processing, memory and executive problems. He then enlarged on each of these to show how a stroke might affect any aspect of cognition. A progress report on the research project 'Work after Stroke' followed (see page 156). There were also practical workshops, and the audience were just as interesting as the speakers. Many people spoke of the support and comradeship they found in the exercise groups. A lady explained how she had heard of the work that Salisbury was doing (see page 72) through the Different Strokes' newsletter and already had an ODFS to help her walk. Now, five years on from her stroke, she was embarking on a device to help her non-functional arm and hand – having had no treatment for them in the intervening years. As she said: '. . . it is only the positive ones like us who get to meetings like this' – we ought to worry about the rest. There were also therapists and researchers, including the team from Glasgow involved in the research study into the needs of younger stroke survivors and their families (see page 156). I got the impression that treatment in Scotland was better than in England. Anyone attending the conference could learn a lot about what can be done for stroke, what is being done and what still needs to be done.

The elderly

In March 2001 the Department of Health published the National Service Framework (NSF) for Older People. To coincide with this the Stroke Association commissioned the College of Health to carry out a large survey of stroke patients and carers. Their findings are reported in *Speaking out about Stroke Services*. Replies to their questionnaire highlighted considerable variability in the perceptions of care available. This report makes disconcerting reading, especially after the previous Stroke Association's report in 1999, *Stroke Care – A Matter of Chance* (see also page 20), following another in 1992. Together they illustrate the lamentably slow rate of improvement in services for the elderly. Perhaps it is misleading to quote only negative comments, but they are most relevant to this age group:

(1) 'I was told by the consultant that my husband was geriatric and therefore did not qualify for intensive therapy.'

(2) 'I'm afraid to say I think I was written off and forgotten.'

(3) 'God help old people on their own with no-one to fight their corner – and believe me fight is the appropriate word.'

Carers also voiced their concerns but, apart from the medical and support needs, what are the priorities for elderly patients? For those, particularly those who live alone, the primary concern will be with mobility and safety. The question always in their minds and those of their families will be whether they will be able to continue with independent living. What help will be available once they are discharged and how will they and their partners – if any – manage?

Professor Kjerstin Ericsson is able to put many issues into a more theoretical framework. She has worked as an associate professor of geriatric nursing in the Department of Neurotec, at the Karolinska Institute, Stockholm, Sweden. Her insights into the more subtle consequences, such as quality of life, perception and neurological neglects, further the aims of this book – to understand stroke. This is aided by her graphic illustrations. Her persective on the personal and economic aspects of home rehabilitation will be thought provoking for those planning stroke services in other countries

Together the three main contributors to this section give a wide perspective to the problems of the different age groups. If I had anything to add it would be to say that whatever the age, health professionals (and carers) should try to project themselves into the mind of the patient. They must try to feel what it is like to be them as they struggle to come to terms with their condition in their particular environment.

CHAPTER 13

Strokes in childhood

DR FENELLA KIRKHAM

STROKE continues to be an important problem in children, affecting at least as many as brain tumour, although with considerably less media attention and health service resources. The perception that nothing can be done is now changing and it is likely that stroke services for young people in general, and children in particular, will improve, so that all can benefit from the ongoing scientific and technological advances. This article outlines the possible causes, necessary investigations and likely treatments for a child with a stroke and emphasises how families can help their own children.

Causes

One of the problems is that there is a very long list of possible causes of stroke, which both doctors and families find very daunting. In fact, most of these are very rare and at least half of children with stroke present 'out-of-the-blue', having never been seriously ill before. World-wide, the commonest cause is sickle cell disease, and in this condition stroke is as common in mid-childhood as it is in elderly adults in general. Cardiac disease is another important cause, although the proportion of children affected has probably fallen as curative surgery has been performed at younger and younger ages, since the risk is almost always reduced after successful operation.

The main thrust of the current research concerns the

cause of stroke in the children for whom it occurs 'out-of-the-blue'. Occasionally a clot may arise from the heart, but this is probably less common than in adults with stroke. Minor injury plays a part in some. There is increasing evidence that infection, e.g. recent chickenpox and recurrent tonsilitis, plays a role; but of course, most children who catch these relatively minor illnesses don't have a stroke. It is likely that those who do, have a predisposition, perhaps genetic, to developing blood vessel narrowing and obstruction when triggered by a common infection. Predispositions might include a tendency to clot more easily or to damage and/or repair the blood vessel much more than average. If the blood vessel wall is narrowed, then a stroke may not happen unless brain tissue is short of oxygen, for example if there is anaemia secondary to iron deficiency or sickle cell disease or hypoxia in a child who is 'blue' because of heart disease or has upper airway obstruction overnight. It is likely that a child with stroke has a combination of risk factors, including a recent trigger, such as trauma or infection, a tendency to relatively sticky blood and some reason for a slightly reduced oxygen supply to the brain tissue.

Tests

When a child presents with acute weakness of one side, one of the first priorities is to establish whether or not there has been bleeding into the brain, which might need surgical removal. CT scanning is a very good method of doing this, although it is not so good at showing if there has been a clot in an artery causing a lack of blood supply to an area of brain (ischaemic stroke), particularly if this is small or if the scan is performed within 24 hours. MRI is better at demonstrating ischaemic stroke, and has the added advantage of being able to show the arteries and veins inside the head. It is now possible to show areas of brain where the blood flow is low but the brain is not yet damaged, and occasionally areas of brain which are very short of oxygen but still capable of surviving. Usually, there is enough information from either a CT or an MRI scan, but occasionally other imaging may be needed such as an arteriogram, a better method of showing the blood vessels, or a single photon emission computed tomography (SPECT) scan, which shows areas of reduced blood flow. The aim is to show whether there is an area of damage and, if so, where; whether there is an abnormality of the blood vessels and, if so, what type, and in some circumstances, whether there is an area of low cerebral blood flow beyond the area of damage.

An echocardiogram (ECHO) is usually performed, to see if there is any structural abnormality e.g. a small hole. A normal electrocardiogram (ECG) excludes the possibility of an abnormal rhythm, which can be associated with clots in the heart breaking off and migrating into the brain circulation, although this is rare in children. A lot of blood is taken, looking for evidence of infection or of a tendency to anaemia or increased blood stickiness or abnormally high lipid levels, e.g. cholesterol. Sometimes specific genetic testing is performed, e.g. for Factor V Leiden which is definitely associated with venous clotting in the legs. A chemical called homocysteine, which is associated with damage to the blood vessel wall if in high concentration, may be measured. Lumbar puncture is often performed, as meningitis is an important cause, and some children with recent chickenpox have abnormal spinal fluid. If there is a history of recurrent tonsillitis or snoring, children may have an overnight sleep study, where oxygen levels are measured, using a small skin probe.

Treatment

If the blood vessel is blocked, the brain tissue beyond it dies after about three hours. It has proved possible, in adults, to unblock the artery and save the brain tissue by using tissue plasminogen activator, but only within a three hour time window; beyond this time there is a high risk of bleeding. It is exceptional for a child to be eligible for this sort of treatment, particularly as it is not appropriate for those who have recently had a procedure, i.e. the majority who stroke in hospital. Emergency transfusion is indicated for children with sickle cell disease who stroke. Occasionally, surgery may be needed, e.g. to remove a large amount of blood or damaged tissue pressing on the brain. For the majority of children, there is nothing that can be done to reduce the amount of damage done at the time of the first stroke and effort is concentrated on preventing further episodes.

Overall, the risk of further stroke is around 10 per cent, but is higher in some groups, e.g. those with sickle cell disease, and lower in others. There is some evidence that genetic predisposition, for example to high homocysteine levels which damage the blood vessel walls, may play a part in encouraging further episodes of blockage, usually in the same blood vessel, but occasionally in others. This is important, as homocysteine can be lowered by increasing the intake of B vitamins, particularly folic acid, vitamin B6 and vitamin B12. For some children, for example those with sickle cell disease, recurrent stroke appears to be related to anaemia and/or hypoxia. Blood transfusion has been to reduce the recurrence risk in this group and oxygen supplementation is under investigation. If the blood vessels are completely blocked, e.g. in Moyamoya (a Japanese term describing the puff of smoke appearance on the arteriogram of the collateral blood vessels attempting to bypass the blockage), then if the blood flow is low, it may be increased after bypass surgery to attach a scalp blood vessel to the blocked one.

Occasionally, it may be appropriate for a child to receive anticoagulation, for example if there is a genetic predisposition to increased blood stickiness, e.g. Factor V Leiden. However, there is a risk of bleeding and patients have to have frequent blood tests. In the majority of children with stroke 'out-of-the-blue', for whom no obvious cause has been found, low dose aspirin (1mg/kg) is prescribed in the medium term, as it has few risks and has been shown to reduce the risk of further strokes in adults. The only way of proving that a treatment is worth taking to reduce the risk of recurrence is to conduct a controlled trial with a large enough number of patients, randomly allocated to one treatment or another or to a placebo.

In addition to specific treatments, changes in lifestyle may reduce the risk of recurrence. It is certainly sensible to eat five portions of fruit or vegetables a day and to take plenty of exercise, e.g. walking to school. Every child should have a balanced diet, with fat and salt-laden foods, e.g. hamburgers and sausages, seen as occasional treats rather than staple foods.

Many children and their parents are devastated by the stroke and anxious about the future. These needs should be met by appropriate professional and lay support.

Making progress

Although many children have a severe weakness of the affected arm and leg immediately after the stroke, the majority make a good recovery and almost all walk, usually with only a minimal limp. Early physiotherapy helps general body movements and occupational therapy usually specif-

TABLE ONE
Common associations with childhood stroke

Children with known illnesses
- Sickle cell disease
- Cardiac disease
- Meningitis
- Immune-deficiency

Previously well children
- Chickenpox
- Recurrent tonsilitis
- Minor head trauma
- Anaemia

Conditions which cause increased blood stickiness
- Factor V Leiden
- Prothrombin 20210
- Increased platelets

Conditions which damage the blood vessel wall
- High homocysteine levels

Abnormal lipids
- Hypercholesterolaemia
- High lipoprotein (a) levels

TABLE TWO
Reducing the risk of recurrence

- Balanced diet: five portions of fruit/vegetables/day
  Fat- and salt-containing foods as treats
- More exercise, e.g. walking to school
- B vitamin supplements: folic acid, B6, B12, Low dose aspirin 1mg/kg/day
- Anti-coagulants for specific circumstances

ically targets hand function. Occasionally children make a good recovery and then develop difficulty in using the affected hand later; this can sometimes be helped by drug treatment or Botulinum toxin injection.

Most children affected by stroke speak as they did before, but occasionally speech therapy is needed. The majority go back into their previous school; it is worthwhile preparing the ground so that teachers know what to expect and most doctors are very happy to prepare an appropriate report. Occasionally children need extra help in school, either with physical challenges, e.g. dressing or in the playground, or with lessons and some of these will need a statement of educational needs.

CHAPTER 14

The specific problems of younger stroke survivors

DONAL O'KELLY

The numbers

Stroke is this country's third biggest killer after cancer and heart disease, and the largest single cause of severe disability. It is commonly seen as an affliction of old age, yet it frequently strikes people in the prime of life, often for no known reason. In the UK, each year over 10,000 people of working age have a stroke – an average of nearly 200 every week. Over 1,000 sufferers are under the age of 30. Recovery can be slow, difficult and sometimes only partial. However, with the right attitude and support, especially in the early stages, dramatic improvements can be made in the quality of life for most stroke survivors. Complete recovery is often possible.

Different Strokes, a charity run by younger stroke sufferers for younger stroke sufferers, recognises the need for a wider choice of services for younger stroke survivors to help them return to a full life and an active role in their community. Stroke survivors have to learn everything from new, slowly moving and improving one day to the next, learning to talk, walk and live again. Different Strokes aims to provide throughout the UK:

- A regional network of exercise classes and swimming sessions (over 24 classes are up and running)

- Practical information packs to survivors
- Access to counselling services
- Benefits and rights information
- Advice and information on education, special training and work opportunities
- A quarterly newsletter to keep members in touch with each other
- Interactive website

The points raised in this section draw directly on Different Strokes' experiences of working with younger stroke survivors, who frequently complain that help currently available has been designed primarily to meet the requirements of older people. Different Strokes advocates a need for a wider choice of services designed for younger stroke survivors, to help them return to a full life and active role in their community.

While in no way wishing to minimise the impact of stroke on older people and their families, Different Strokes suggests that the needs of a 20-year-old stroke survivor will be quite different to those of someone aged 80, not least because the 20-year-old is faced not just by years but, hopefully, decades over which to recover from stroke and cope with its impact on family, education, work and social relationships. Rehabilitation, therefore, must be planned carefully and appropriately to maximise the potential of younger stroke survivors to return to independent living. Different Strokes believes that addressing the following issues would facilitate this process and at the same time contribute to reducing long term dependence on health and social services.

The anecdotal nature of some of these issues is acknowledged but, in the absence of formal research evidence on younger stroke patients, it is hoped it may generate discussion on the needs of this important, but often ignored, group of patients.

The wish list

At the first onset of stroke, we want to be believed. We have often heard examples of people being treated by health professionals who appear not to understand that stroke can affect young people, with symptoms ascribed to other conditions, from migraine to being drunk.

We want to be looked after by staff who understand our specific needs. Specialised stroke nurses on dedicated stroke units would be a good start.

Younger adults with stroke often report distress at being admitted to and cared for on elderly care wards. Greater consideration needs to be given to the appropriate setting and location for the care and early rehabilitation of younger stroke patients while in hospital.

We want staff to be aware of, and address, not only the physical effects of stroke but also its emotional, social and psychological impact. Consideration should be given to providing/improving access to counselling to help younger stroke survivors come to terms and deal with both the short-term effect of stroke but also help us adjust to its long-term implications for housing, personal finances, education and employment.

At discharge from hospital, we do not want to be 'written off' as disabled. We want a long-term plan of care which recognises that we are embarking on a slow but gradual recovery.

Existing discharge advice and information is designed to meet the needs of older people. Information on long-term care or nursing homes, for example, is usually not relevant to the needs of younger stroke survivors who want discharge advice tailored to their own specific short- and longer-term needs and circumstances. The bingo and basket-weaving currently available at the local day-centre is not always appropriate!

The goals of most younger stroke survivors include achieving, as far as possible, a gradual return to independent living, to employment and re-integration into family and social life. Those who design and provide services need to recognise that these goals may differ from those of older people and tailor rehabilitation services accordingly. Emphasis needs to be on treating the patients as individuals, taking age and personal factors into account.

After discharge, the transitional nature of recovery from stroke means that we should have an open-ended commitment to ongoing monitoring and assessment of our recovery so that rehabilitation services meet our needs appropriately as they change over time. This could be facilitated by ensuring that, as patients, we have details of a specific person who can be contacted to organise re-assessment of our needs as we progress in our recovery.

In meeting the goals of younger stroke survivors, rehabilitation services need to address the specific issues of re-education, retraining and re-employment.

Recognising that existing health and social services cannot meet the full range of ongoing and long-term rehabilitation needs of younger stroke survivors, consideration should be given to developing innovative ways of meeting some of these needs. Models such as GP schemes for prescribing exercise, opportunities for using leisure centres, etc. merit further investigation.

Younger stroke survivors have a range of information needs, including general advice on disability and help on getting aids and gadgets; information on benefits, social services and patients rights; applying to charities for individual grants; coping with the psychological impact of stroke and people's attitudes to stroke; advice on sex and relationships (notes on these topics are produced by Different Strokes). NHS purchasers and providers should ensure that younger stroke survivors have timely access to these or comparable leaflets.

A number of organisations can provide advice on the specific issue of helping people with disabilities back to work. Health professionals in primary, community and secondary care need to be aware of the different organisations that can help younger stroke survivors, and need to convey this information to these younger survivors in systematic and timely ways.

Carers of people with stroke have their own support, advice and information needs. Special consideration needs to be given to address the needs of carers of younger stroke survivors, taking into account both the possible long-term nature of this caring role and its transitional and variable nature over time.

The hidden side of stroke

In younger people a stroke happens suddenly. It is a traumatic and devastating experience. We are somewhere in the course of our daily life when it strikes – at work, on holiday, relaxing at home, socialising with friends, or even asleep. Wherever we are, or whatever we are doing, our lives are brought to a complete standstill. Because many of us have had no previous experience of severe illness, the devastating effects of stroke are even more difficult to deal with. Stroke is about loss. The sudden loss of a fully functioning body and mind which we have always taken for granted.

Now, instead, we have paralysed arms and legs, an inability to speak or be understood, incontinence, lack of concentration, poor vision, no short-term memory, uncontrollable laughter or tears, or any combination of the above and more. We find it very hard to relate to ourselves as 'ill' people, let alone disabled in some way.

Possibly, we have never been in hospital before, but almost certainly we will now experience hospitalisation and/or rehabilitation units, usually for weeks or even months. We are removed from life, work, relationships, friends and leisure time and become institutionalised as we begin the long, slow and difficult process of rehabilitation. Anyone who has had a stroke will know about the huge changes that it brings about. The loss of the freedom to 'get on with life' whilst the rest of the world goes by. We are not allowed to function as before but are left feeling vulnerable, helpless, without dignity, frightened and isolated.

This is the invisible side of stroke. No one can see those feelings, or those thoughts. Others can only see the sudden functional loss of parts of our body and, of course, it is vital that we work as hard as possible to regain as much as we can of what we have physically lost. However, it is equally vital that we allow ourselves to consider the 'invisible side of stroke'. It is not only our bodies which have been damaged, but our thoughts and feelings too. It is totally impossible to have a stroke and not experience extremes of emotion, fear and anxiety about life, work, family and close relationships, but most of all emotions about our relationship with, and perception of, ourselves. Everything changes after a stroke and everyone's recovery is individual. The most vital thing is that we give ourselves the very best chance of getting better.

It is not easy to ignore the physical changes which a

stroke causes, but it is easy to ignore the 'invisible' ones. Acknowledging them and facing them can give us a fuller, more rounded recovery.

Different Strokes offers an opportunity to talk over the phone, or to meet with other stroke survivors at regular exercise classes. This will give you a chance to share your experiences with other people who have suffered similar loss themselves. It can help to remove the sense of isolation which having a stroke so often causes.

Different Strokes: Telephone number: 08451 307172
Website: www.differentstrokes.co.uk
Email: different@strokes.demon.co.uk

CHAPTER 15

Some issues in stroke management for the elderly

PROFESSOR KJERSTIN ERICSSON

STROKE, referred to as apoplexy in Greek literature, has been recognised since ancient times. Hippocrates, about 400BC, described apoplexy, and it is perceived as particularly common in older people. The World Health Organisation (WHO) has defined stroke as 'rapidly developing signs of focal disturbance of cerebral function, with symptoms lasting 24 hours or longer or leading to death, with no apparent cause other than of vascular origin' (WHO, 1971). In years gone by, stroke patients finished their days in institutions with no possibility of influencing how they lived their own lives. Today, new techniques and treatments have made it possible for stroke patients to have an early discharge and to continue their treatment and training at home. This chapter concentrates on some issues involved in stroke rehabilitation that are presumed to be of utmost importance in enabling stroke patients to live independently in society. Parts that will be highlighted upon are quality of life, activity and mobility, perception, communication and social support, caring and the situation of the relatives, and home rehabilitation versus rehabilitation in an institution.

Stroke and quality of life

It is to be expected that a stroke will, at least temporarily, affect the patient's quality of life and may lead to varying degrees of depression. Quality of life (QoL) is a subjective concept used in all kind of situations, not least in health care. When something important occurs, like a stroke, the concept of QoL can, despite or perhaps because of its subjectivity, be a conclusive measure of all the experiences of life. The more dependent the patients are, the worse the quality of their life is likely to be.

QoL in some way depends on how well a patient manages practical activities in daily living (ADL). All kind of aids, either human or technical, that can compensate for reduced possibilities to independence can increase the QoL. Persistent motor impairment and ADL-disability in stroke patients sometimes produces long-lasting negative effects on several aspects of life satisfaction, in the sexual and leisure domains, for instance. The level of social well-being after stroke can be seen as a consequence of the adequacy of the coping ability process (Viitanen et al., 1988).

Stroke patients rate their health, and especially their emotions and feelings of social isolation, as much worse than that of people of similar age. Stroke patients' QoL has been measured in many different ways. The 'Nottingham Health Profile' (NHP) is a questionnaire designed to measure social and personal effects of illness on well-being. Ebrahim et al (1986) found through the NHP that many patients experienced pain, were emotionally distressed, had disturbed sleep, poor mobility, and were socially isolated. These are important, potentially treatable problems, not usually considered in the management of stroke patients. However, many of the patients did not have contact with either their GP or any other person or source of help. The pain from arthritis was also a contributing factor to patients putting more weight on the unaffected side. One conclusion of the study was that, when evaluating stroke rehabilitation outcome, it is important not only to rely on an ADL assessment, but to include an indicator of QoL. Improved physical ability may not always mean improved self-perceived health.

A study from Sweden (Jadback, 1993) investigated why some stroke patients experienced good quality of life and some did not. Quality of life was defined as the patients' own evaluation of the content of their life. The results could differentiate between low and high scoring QoL. The patients with high QoL were characterised by good ADL capacity. This was the best predictor to the experience of life two years after stroke. Stroke patients with no remaining symptoms like paresis or speech difficulties will be assumed to be recovered. They will be expected to be happy and satisfied with their outcome or condition. Screening these patients, however, often reveals one or several problems. Seven out of ten were reported having a lowered QoL compared with their peer group. When a negative change of the QoL has been found, it is essential that professional help is sought to find the reason, because it can be a sign of an ongoing depression. It was noted that 50 per cent of the patients were depressed and worried, and that, without really having a serious handicap. It was concluded that the depression and the worries *per se*, caused the low QoL, and that impaired circulation in the brain often gives depressive reactions.

Depression

Depressive reactions can be different according to the stage of the stroke. It was found that in the acute phase the risk factor was a frontal left-sided lesion. Reduced ability to manage on their own and speech difficulties became the two most important risk factors to having a depression three months after the stroke. One year after the stroke it was a poor social support that caused most of the depressive symptoms (Bernspång, 1997).

QUESTION 10. WELLBEING

Where are you on this hill? (tick one circle)

MEN

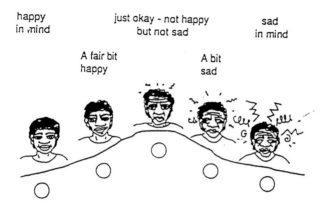

WOMEN

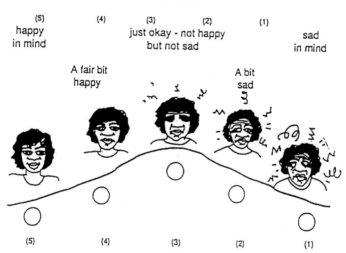

An adaptation of the delighted-terrible (D-T) face scale (Holmén et al, 2000), for use in Australia with aborigines.

Detecting and assessing depression

Different instruments can be used to detect and assess depression. If the patient can participate in an ordinary questionnaire there are many well-established instruments, for example Montgomery & Asberg (1979). However, many patients in the acute phase of a stroke are very tired. Others have speech difficulties, so interviewing them poses practical problems. For these patients there needs to be a rapid and easy way of testing their mood. One old, useful instrument is the delighted-terrible (D–T) face scale. It was first elaborated by Andrew-Withey (1976) to study well-being in elderly Americans.

The delighted-terrible (D-T) face scale, first elaborated by Andrew-Withey to study well-being in elderly Americans.

Patients have only to mark which face most closely corresponds to their mood. This has also been used in Stockholm, Sweden, for elderly stroke patients who were unable to talk (Murray, unpublished paper). In Australia, where it was also used, the faces were modified when used with aborigines (Holmén et al., 2000).

It has also been used to detect so-called masked depressions. Those have no detectable influence on the mood, but show through changes of temperament, appetite, strength or sleep patterns from one day to the next. In Stockholm the nurses used to talk with each patient for several minutes when giving out medicine. Then they asked the questions: 'How has your day been since yesterday in relation to temperament, strength, sleep and appetite? Please indicate

with a cross, improvement, deterioration, or no change.'
They were given a simple chart like the one below.

Var snäll och besvara dessa åtta frågor varje kväll och svara precis som Din upplevelse har varit.˙

1. Hur uppskattar Du din smärta idag?

Ingen smärta --- Outhärdlig smärta

2. Tog inte extra smärtlindrande☐   Haft telefonkontakt med ASIH för smärtproblematik☐

Tog extra smärtlindrande☐   Haft hembesök av ASIH för smärtproblematik☐

3. Om Du kände oro – ängslan eller rädsla idag hur mycket uppskattar Du den till?

Inget -- Outhärdligt

4 a. Hur har Du upplevt din smärtlindring idag?

4 b. Hur har Du upplevt ditt humör idag?

4 c. Hur har Du upplevt din ork idag?

4 d. Hur har Du upplevt aptiten idag?

4 e. Hur har Du upplevt sömnen natten som var?

Avemark & Ericsson 1999 ©

Chart used by nurses in Stockholm to help detect masked depressions.

Another study used the same questions but with the D–T scale. It was performed in palliative care of cancer patients in the terminal stage. This was done to optimise the information with the least possible effort on the part of the patients (Avemark et al., 2000). An Australian paper focused on possible risk factors other than the site of lesion in the brain. It found that functional impairment, living in a nursing home, and being divorced were significantly associated with post-stroke depression. No such associations were found to age, sex, social class, cognitive impairment or pre-stroke physical illness (Burvill et al., 1997).

A real depression after stroke has to be treated with anti-depressive drugs. The treatment itself can hasten the general recovery in all areas, physical as well as mental. It can have beneficial effects on paresis, aphasia, and ability to manage on your own, as well as on the ability to concentrate and the memory capacity. In this way the QoL will also be improved. How can this be? Perhaps it is due to the anti-depressive effect. When a patient does not suffer from the 'heavy' mood related to the depression, or problems with taking initiative, it will become easier to benefit from ordinary rehabilitation. There is also speculation that the treatment could have direct effect on the brain lesion in the sense that it can recover faster or trigger compensation mechanisms.

Perception

One of the more distressing manifestations of stroke impairment affects the perceptual field. That means how the patients perceive themselves and their environment. One aspect of the impairment is visual (recognition of colours, forms, and body details). A further aspect is more complex, and includes the perception of situations. This type of perception demands an active participation from the patient. It concerns the understanding of how a pattern is built up, and how to reconstruct another one (Bernspång, 1997). This means, that it might be difficult to draw a house, tree, or person.

This type of perceptual impairment can be tested by human figure drawing (HFD), copying geometrical figures, or by drawing the clock test. For the clock test, patients are asked to draw the clock face by heart, and to indicate the time given, by putting the numbers and hands on the clock face.

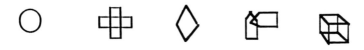

Geometric figures to test certain types of perceptual impairment.
Ericsson K, Forssell L G,Holmén K, Viitanem M, Winblad B. (1996)

The practical implications are not being able to, or having the difficulties when trying to, recognise objects. This can cause problems for stroke patients. They may not be able to find what they are looking for or understand what they see in the environment. This also means that it may be difficult to separate objects from their background. For instance they might not see the towel put on the bed, the cup in the cupboard, or the toothbrush in the holder. Stroke patients can find it difficult, even in their own home, to locate the kitchen when they are in the next room. Even approaching something familiar from a different direction, for instance coming out of the tube from an unusual exit, can cause the stroke patient to feel lost, be distressed and even to break down because they may not be able to handle such a situation.

141

Impaired distance judgement is another common perceptual problem. At home this might mean falling over furniture, crashing into doors. A near invisible glass on a table is likely to get broken as a result of misjudged distance. It can also be difficult to differentiate between the top and bottom, or front and back, of an object. This means it might be difficult to handle a tool that has a special function.

Neurological neglects

A neglect means a dysfunction or inability of patients to respond or orientate themselves to stimuli in space (spatial unilateral neglect) or presented to one-half of the body (personal unilateral neglect), the side opposite to the one affected by the stroke (Tham, 1998). Unilateral neglect (UN) refers to patients ignoring their left hemispace. The term was first presented 125 years ago by Jackson (1876). Mesulam defined the UN as being 'not a deficit of seeing, hearing, feeling, or moving but one of looking, listening, touching, and searching' (Mesulam, 1985 p.142).

Neglect is a result of the stroke patient's brain not having registered information from a certain part of the body and the corresponding part of the environment. The left side is most often affected, but it may occur also after left-sided lesions.

The person in question is not always aware of his problems, or does not understand or even realise that anything is wrong. Even if it is obvious to any outside observer that something is very wrong the patient can not comprehend. When told, patients most likely might shrug their shoulders, and try to provide what to them is a plausible, but to others a bizarre, explanation. Spontaneous recovery takes place in most patients within a few weeks after the stroke (Hier et al., 1983). In practice, neglect means that it is impossible to locate an object; when it is placed it is placed to the left side, if that is the side from which the patient can no longer register the input. Likewise, patients can eat everything placed to the right side of the plate, neglecting the left side; they dress only one side and not the other, and they read only text written on the right hand side of the page if the lesion is on the left side. If they have to draw or write, they easily 'forget' to draw parts of the figure on one side. Not getting information from one side of the body also means not being motivated to move any part of this side of the body.

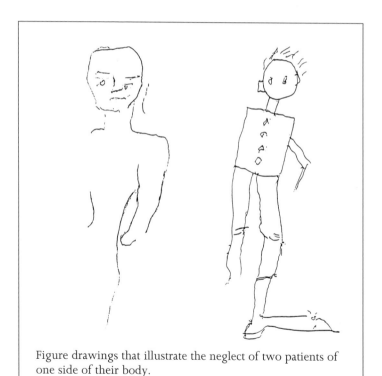

Figure drawings that illustrate the neglect of two patients of one side of their body.

Activity and mobility

Maintaining balance while standing depends on the integration of sensory inputs (somatic, visual, and vestibular) with the motor processes in the limbs and trunk. Most elderly people have to concentrate more to maintain posture. Even healthy elderly persons have a reduced central capacity, resulting in increased reaction time. This is still more accentuated in cerebrovascular accidents like strokes, where the postural information is reduced (Overstall, 1995). Patients have a tendency to weightbear asymmetrically when standing upright. This is because they misjudge the vertical, and horizontal sensory inputs.

The leg muscles are more impaired than the trunk and they are critical to moving the body mass over the base of support. The stance after stroke is usually asymmetric with about 70 per cent of the total body weight shifted on to the unaffected leg. In this way the postural sway is increased. The more unsteady the stance – the more it affects the walking pattern. The gait in a hemiplegia is characterised by slower and shorter steps, lack of smoothness and asymmetry. Another study concentrated on improved gait balance, muscle strength and modified environments. It showed that these three factors reduced the risk of falling by 30 per cent (Overstall, 1995).

The ability to balance while reaching for a variety of objects, both within and beyond arm's length, has been reported to be critical to independent living. After a stroke many patients also have difficulties keeping their balance when seated. Sitting balance has been shown to be useful as a prognostic indicator of the outcome of the disease. This study also showed that stroke patients, specially trained in sitting balance, improved faster and achieved more (Dean & Shepherd, 1997). A task-related motor training is thus efficient in improving the ability of balance while seated, and one of the goals of stroke rehabilitation.

From an activity and mobility perspective the aim is to start the motor training while still in hospital. Motivation is the key to success. Then the patient should be encouraged to take up such previously practised motor activities as are possible. If this is not possible other activities need to be established. Together with technical aids and home equipment much can be done to improve the patient's home situation. These tasks are common to the activity and mobility perspective. Treating cognitive difficulties in the ADL-situation requires the co-operation and participation of both patient and carer. The patients may need to be even more motivated than others and that can be achieved by letting them choose the activity in question to be trained. Relatives must be informed and comprehend the implications of the cognitive dysfunction.

Physiotherapists have specific tasks in the mobility training, such as trying to get the patient to recognise obstacles as well as the possibilities in the home environment. Also it is important that the patient and relative are prepared to take some risks. That means daring to do certain tasks when the capacity exists, when they are not too dangerous. The ultimate aim is to reach the highest possible level of independence by identifying and training the necessary skills. Mobility rehabilitation is primarily directed towards specific motor functions, such as standing, walking, keeping the balance, in order to optimise the independence of the patient. Indirectly it is also advantageous for the care giver. This is achieved by using walking aids, learning to manage stairs and finally being able to venture outside the home. However, it is not always easy to persuade the patient to co-operate .

Communication and social support

Another very important perspective is that of communication, where especially the aphasic stroke patients can profit from the help of speech therapists. Amongst stroke patients, 20–33 per cent of those needing continued rehabilitation have aphasic problems. It is unusual that speech therapy is taken into consideration when talking about home rehabilitation. The aphasics (patients with language, speech, and verbal impairments) and those with cognitive difficulties constitute a qualitatively different group to those having only motor problems. Therapists often have to explain, prepare and solve these problems with patients and those near to them, and, if necessary, they function as interpreter. These difficulties can make the transfer of information, as well as the motivation, more difficult, and may necessitate a longer period of speech therapy. Aphasic patients need help to formulate their own aims for verbal and psychosocial improvement.

The social perspective bridges the gap between the hospital and the home rehabilitation team. The social support should begin before discharge by preparing and counselling the relatives. Welfare officers are the social experts in any home rehabilitation team, individually informing patients and relatives about stroke and the societal support. The social network surrounding patients is of great significance to their life satisfaction. This network decreases with age, and leads to an increasing feeling of loneliness.

From the perspective of relatives and carers

A second perspective is that of caring, characterised in concentrating on transmission of knowledge to the home service staff concerning the stroke patient, and his/her problems with stomach, intestines (constipation) and incontinence. They may need advice about taking medication and any after-effects, as well as eating and drinking problems. Cognitively impaired stroke patients have even more difficulties in getting advantage from any treatment and probably need more help than others.

Relatives play an important role in the life of the stroke patient. When working with perceptual impairment and aphasia they must not forget that the patient is the same person as before, so should be treated as such. Talk to patients, not about them or over their heads. The best way of helping them is by encouraging them in as many previous activities as possible. Facilitate really difficult tasks for them, but do not do everything for them. Striving and achieving anything difficult can only be beneficial. Give support and comfort. It is important for stroke patients to feel that they can manage certain tasks and situations even if it takes a long time. But caring is wearing and it is important that carers look after their own health.

The advantages of home rehabilitation

The home rehabilitation team (HRT) performs a 'bridging' function, starting the training in hospital, continuing after release to the patient's own home. The aim of the rehabilitation is to optimise the independence not only of the stroke patient but also indirectly of the family. However, not all patients appreciate the invasion of care givers into their home. Thus it is highly important to respect the individual's integrity, when working as the HRT do.

The development of methods of treatment and the organisation of cost-effective stroke rehabilitation have always been, and are still today, challenges to the health care systems. The stroke patient group is already large because the incidence of stroke increases with age. It will increase in the future with the increasing number of elderly in the society. The rehabilitation will prove very expensive and put considerable burden on society. How to organise rehabilitation to achieve an optimal result is open to debate. One point in question is the length of time a stroke patient should be treated in hospital. The time spent in acute hospital and rehabilitation wards is tending to decrease, and in many countries it is questioned whether all stroke patients need to be admitted at all (Burnard, 1988; Mulley & Arie, 1978). An alternative to in-patient care would be day care, polyclinic treatment, or home rehabilitation.

The purpose of home rehabilitation is to maintain a person in his chosen environment, usually his own home. Some patients are too disabled to be at home in the early stages in their treatment. In home rehabilitation many professional groups are involved in teamwork and their special tasks include:

- decreasing the risk of depression, thus increasing quality of life (QoL) after discharge

- helping patient and relative to feel more comfortable with care and rehabilitation

- giving patient and relative better information, and becoming more implicated in planning for the discharge

- improving communication between hospital, home service and home rehabilitation team, even before discharge

- minimising the length of stay in hospital.

The team members all have their own field of responsibility. They represent different perspectives such as activities, not only ADL but also personal to the patient, also mobility, social contacts, communication, and direct caring (Milton et al., 1996).

Home rehabilitation has many advantages over out-patient treatment. The fatigue caused by travelling can then be avoided and the patient can wholly profit from the planned training (Partridge, 1987). Frail patients can avoid the awkwardness of transferring. Finally transport can be difficult to organise, can involve a lot of waiting about or even missing appointments.

Suitable training at home can take into consideration the life style and the motivation of the patient and all concerned (Burnard, 1988; Kavanagh, 1971; Wade & Langton Hewer, 1983). Moreover, treatment is often more effective and more efficient if given at home (Stone, 1987; Glossop & Smith, 1981; Boyd, 1987). The role of the relative is of importance to the outcome of the rehabilitation (Evans et al., 1994). If the relatives have a realistic attitude to difficulties and an understanding of what can be achieved, this is just as important as the patient's own attitude. In fact it can be a prerequisite for optimal outcome. The reduced cost of home rehabilitation is another argument in its favour, being far less than in institutions, despite being equally effective (Young & Forster, 1991, 1992, 1993; Gladman et al., 1994; Gladman & Lincoln, 1994).

References

Avemark C, Ericsson K. 'Gender differences in experienced pain, mood, energy, appetite and sleep by cancer patients in palliative care' (submitted).

Bernspang B. 'Perception och hur den kan forandras vid stroke', (Perception and how it can be changed in case of stroke), Stockholm: Riksforbundet mot hjarnans karlsjukdomar13p (in Swedish), 1997.

Boyd RV. 'The rehabilitation of stroke illness', *The Practitioner*, 23, 1987, pp. 890–5.

Burnard S. 'Development pf a community physiotherapy service', *Physiotherapy*, 1988, 74, pp. 4–8.

Burvill P, Johnson G, Jamrozik K, Anderson C, & Stewart-Wynne E. 'Risk factors for post-stroke depression', *International Journal of Geriatric Psychiatry*, 12, pp. 219–26.

Ebrahim S, Barer D, & Nouri F. 'Use of the Nottingham Health Profile with patients after a stroke', *Journal of Epidemiology and Community Health*, 198), 40, pp. 166–9.

Ericsson K, Forssell L G,Holmén K, Viitanem M, Winblad B. 'Copying and handwriting ability in the screening of cognitive dysfunction in old age', *Arch Gerontol Geriatr*, 22, pp. 103–121.

Evans R L, Connis R T, Bishop D S, Hendricks R D, Haselkorn J K. 'Stroke: a family dilemma', *Disability and Rehabilitation*, 1994, 16(3), 110–18.

Gladman J R F, & Lincoln N. 'Follow-up of a controlled trial of domiciliary stroke rehabilitation' (DOMINO study), *Age and Ageing*, 1994, 23, pp. 9–13.

Gladman J R F, Whynes D, & Lincoln N. 'Cost comparison of domiciliary and hospital-based stroke rehabilitation', *Age and Ageing*, 1994, 23, pp. 241–5.

Glossop E S, & Smith D S. 'Domiciliary physiotherapy research project 1976–8'. *Physiotherapy*, 1981, 67, pp. 79–.

Hier D B, Mondlock J, & Caplan L R. 'Recovery of behaviour abnormalities after right hemisphere stroke', Neurology, 1983, 33, pp. 345–50.

Holmén K, Ekstrom U, Senior K. 'Loneliness amongst Elderly Aboriginal Persons Living in an Aged Care Centre for Aboriginal People' (Submitted).

Jackson J H. 'Case of large cerebral tumour without optic neuritis and with left hemiplegia and imperception', Royal Ophtalmical Hospital Reports, 1876, 8, pp. 434–44.

Jadback G. 'Livskvalitet efter stroke' (Quality of life after stroke), Sjukskotersketidningen, 1993, (7), pp. 216–18.

Katz S, Ford A B, Moskowitz R W, Jackson B A, & Jaffe M W. 'Studies of illness in the aged: The index of ADL: A standardized measure of biological and sociobiological function', Journal of American Medical Association, 1963, 185, pp. 914–19.

Kavanagh T. 'Home and outpatient rehabilitation: A two-year comparative study', Canadian Medical Association Journal, 1971, 105, pp. 65–9.

Lovgren B. 'Rehabilitation of old people with stroke. Outcome prediction and long-term follow-up' Doctoral Dissertation from the Department of Community Medicine and Rehabilitation, Division of Geriatric Medicine, Umeå University, Sweden.

Mesulam M M. 'Attention, confusional states and neglect', In: M M Mesulam (Ed.). Principles of behavioural neurology, 1985, pp. 125–68, Philadelphia:Davis Company.

Milton A, Gustafsson D, Liljeqvist A, Wall B, & Lokk J. 'Allt I hemmet – Hemrehabilitering av strokerehabilitering'. (Everything at home – home rehabilitation of stroke patients). Report from Division of Geriatric Medicine, Huddinge University Hospital, Stockholm, Sweden, 1966.

Montgomery S A, & Åsberg M. 'A new depression scale designed to be sensitive to change', British Journal of Psychiatry, 1979, 134, pp. 382–9.

Mulley G, & Arie T. 'Treating stroke: Home or hospital?' British Medical Journal 1978, (2), pp. 1321–2.

Murray V. 'Depression och livskvalitet efter stroke', (Depression and quality of life after stroke) Stockholm: Riksforbundet mot hjarnans karlsjukdomar13p (in Swedish), 1997.

Nydevik I. 'Stroke in geriatric patients. Functional ability and need for care', *Doctoral Dissertation from the Department of Clinical Neuroscience and Family Medicine, Section of Geriatric Medicine*, Karolinska Institutet, Stockholm, Sweden, 1994.

Overstall P W. 'Falls after stroke', *British Medical Journal*, 1995, 8; 311 (6997): pp. 74–5.

Partridge C. 'Physiotherapy in the community', *Journal of Royal College of General Practicians*, 1987, 37, pp. 194–5.

Stone M. 'Physiotherapy support to a domiciliary care scheme for physically handicapped elderly people', *Physiotherapy*, 1987, 73, pp. 227–9.

Tham K. 'Unilateral neglect: Aspects of rehabilitation from an occupational therapy perspective', *Doctoral Dissertation from the Department of Neurotec, division of Occupational Therapy*, Karolinska Institutet, Stockholm, Sweden, 1998.

Viitanen M, Fugl-Meyer K, Bernspång B, & Fugl-Meyer A. 'Life satisfaction in long term survivors after stroke', *Scandinavian Journal of Rehabilitation Medicine*, 1988, 20, pp. 17–24.

Wade D T, & Langton Hewer R. 'Why admit stroke patients to hospital?' *The Lancet*, 1983, i, pp. 807–9.

World Health Organisation. 'Cerebrovascular diseases. Prevention, treatment and rehabilitation', *Geneve: World Health Organisation*, 1971.

Young J B, & Forster A. 'Methodology of a stroke rehabilitation trial', *Clinical Rehabilitation*, 1991, 5, pp. 127–33.

Young J B, & Forster A. 'The Bradford community stroke trial: results at six months', *British Medical Journal*, 304, 1992, pp. 1085–9.

Young J B, & Forster A. 'Day hospital and home physiotherapy for stroke patients: a comparative cost-effectiveness study', *Journal of the Royal College of Physiology*, London, 1993, 27, pp. 252–8.

Part 4

RESEARCH

CHAPTER 16

An introduction to research

THE WHOLE of this book is some kind of crescendo – progressing from the mainly anecdotal via the advisory to the academic. The first part of the book does not include references, but the referenced content builds up in the next sections. Research is being undertaken at many different levels all round the world. This introduction gives the general reader an idea of some projects sponsored by charitable foundations in Great Britain.

The Stroke Association

The Stroke Association is the only charity exclusively concerned with research into stroke. From the extensive list of the projects it has funded in the past few years several have direct bearing on parts of this book, and just a few are listed:

National Childhood Stroke Survey. Dr A N Williams, Springfields Medical Centre, The Birmingham Children's Hospital, Selly Oak, Birmingham B29 6JB

A Study to Evaluate the Met and Unmet Needs of Young Stroke Survivors. Professor D L McLellan, Dr Ann Ashburn, Dr Paula Kersten, and Dr S George, Rehabilitation Research Unit, Southampton General Hospital, Tremona Road, Southampton SO16 6YD

Randomised Controlled Trial to Test the Efficiency of Manual Acupuncture for Recovery of Balance and Activities of Daily Living after Stroke. Dr A R White and Dr M James, Department of Complementary Medicine, University of Exeter, 25 Victoria Park Road, Exeter EX2 4NT

Cognitive Rehabilitation Using Response Guided Errorless Learning With Stroke Patients. Prof G Humphreys, Prof A Wing, Dr R M Bracewell, and Dr Bonnie Connor, School of Psychology, University of Birmingham, Edgbaston, Birmingham B15 2TT

A full list of the numerous research projects funded by the Stroke Association can be found on their website.

Other charitable trusts

The Joseph Rowntree Foundation has supported Connect (see page 96), which is a charity for those with aphasia, in their work, funding the research and production for their publications *Talking about Aphasia*, and the *Aphasia Handbook*. At present they are also supporting Connect's project into what happens to patients with severe aphasia when they try to adapt to life after a stroke: what it is like and what are the implications for daily life for them and those around them. At the same time the Medical Research Council is supporting their work into inclusive intellectual access.

Different Strokes received a grant from The National Lottery to fund research into the barriers that prevent stroke survivors getting back to work. Entitled 'Work after Stroke' the research is being carried out by Professor Karen Bryan at the European Institute of Health and Medical Sciences, University of Surrey.

The Chest Heart & Stroke Scotland is funding a study into 'The Needs of Younger Stroke Survivors and their Families'. This research is being carried out by Strathclyde Centre for Disability Research, University of Glasgow, and The Physical Disability Research Unit, Southern General Hospital, Glasgow.

Action Research is a medical research charity that has, in the past twenty years, funded 36 projects related to stroke. At present they are supporting a research project at the William Harvey Hospital, Ashford, Kent into the problems of swallowing after stroke and silent aspiration.

Research into Ageing is at present funding a programme at Keele University into the relationships between sensory and motor functions and their role in recovery of hand function following stroke. The researcher, a physiotherapist, has a particular interest in the effects and effectiveness of therapy for stroke patients specifically regarding the upper limb and hand.

The next and final chapter, contributed by the team from the Behavioural Brain Sciences Centre, the University of Birmingham, is based on work sponsored by the Stroke Association. It explains how experimental psychologists organise and prepare their research into cognitive rehabilitation.

CHAPTER 17

Response-guided learning: research in cognitive rehabilitation*

BONNIE B CONNOR, DELROY A HARVEY, R MARTYN
BRACEWELL, GLYN W HUMPHREYS AND ALAN M WING

Introduction

Stroke is the leading cause of severe disability in England
and Wales (Stroke Association, 2001) and in the United
States (National Stroke Association, 2001). Additionally,
stroke is increasingly being recognized in children. In adults,
as in children, the increased incidence of disability is directly
related to the increased survival rate. For adults, more are
surviving strokes and, for children, more are surviving the
previously fatal conditions predisposing them to stroke,
such as congenital heart disease, sickle cell anaemia, and
leukemia (deVeber G, Roach E S, Riela A R, Wiznitzer M,
2000). Whether adult or child, two-thirds of stroke survivors have moderate to severe impairments. The indirect
costs of stroke in adults includes billions of pounds in lost
productivity annually. For children there are the increased
costs of providing education that adequately addresses their
physical and cognitive needs.

Age is a known risk factor for stroke, with the incidence
of stroke doubling in each decade after the age of 55. This
post-WW II 'baby boom' generation of over-50-year-olds is

* This research was supported by a grant from the Stroke Association
(UK). We acknowledge the assistance of Wittenstein Aktiv Technologies Ltd in the provision of equipment for the research.

expected to rise by 19 per cent between 1994 and 2000, placing more people at higher risk for stroke daily (Dobkin, 1998). This increase in risk for stroke, coupled with the increased survival rate following stroke, raises the likelihood that more people will be living longer with moderate to severe disability.

Disability can be physical, cognitive, or both. The most obvious physical disability following stroke is hemiparesis, paralysis of one side of the body, with the arm usually being weaker than the leg. More subtle, but potentially far more disruptive to normal daily activities, is the presence of cognitive deficits. The incidence of cognitive deficits following stroke has been estimated to be greater than 35 per cent (Tatemichi et al., 1994). These deficits appear as disruptions to normal functions of attention, perception, thinking, learning, and memory. For example, the stroke survivor may have difficulty, while in hospital or during out-patient therapy, learning the names of his therapists and then remembering them from one appointment to the next.

There are also definite differences in the types of cognitive problems, depending on where in the brain the stroke damage occurred. The types of cognitive problems experienced by someone with damage to the left side of the brain can be quite different from damage to the right side. With left-sided brain damage, hemiparesis will be on the right side of the body, and cognitive problems will often have to do with language and 'praxis' – the ability to do skilled movements, particularly in their proper sequence. The language problems may affect the patient's ability to comprehend (receptive aphasia) or the ability to communicate (expressive aphasia), or both (global aphasia). Damage on the right side of the brain will affect movement of the left side of the body and is more often accompanied by problems of attention and

159

spatial perception. A common disorder of attention and perception is referred to as 'unilateral spatial neglect'. A person with this condition has a tendency to fail to attend to the side of space opposite the side of the brain that is damaged. They will show a tendency for decreased or absent awareness of events presented to that half of the body. Though there is not necessarily any problem with their vision, they may fail to complete the left hand side of drawings or to eat food from the left side of the plate, and they may not respond to commands from the left side of space. They may even fail to recognize the limbs on the left hand side as their own (Riddoch & Humphreys, 1983). Cueing attention to the affected side can help, suggesting that there is a problem in attending to that side of space.

Several studies have shown that patients with these types of attentional deficits are significantly more impaired in their activities of daily living (ADLs) than patients with no attentional deficits. We also know that cognitive impairment following stroke results in poorer rehabilitation outcomes (Jeffery & Good, 1995), decreased quality of life (Kwa, Limburg, & deHaan, 1996; Riddoch, Humphreys, & Bateman, 1995), and increased incidence of depression (Starkstein & Robinson 1990). The focus of neuropsychological rehabilitation, whether with stroke patients or other types of brain injury, is to reduce the everyday consequences of impaired cognitive functioning (disability) and the extent to which these problems interfere with successful return to society (level of handicap) (Wilson, 1998a).

One of the most remarkable aspects of the brain is its ability to 'repair itself' following injury, a capability referred to as neuroplasticity. This does not necessarily mean that the brain generates new brain cells in the same way that the skin would develop new skin cells to heal a cut. What it does mean is that areas of the brain that previously were dedicated to one particular function may take on additional functions, much like a work group in which a number of people have been made redundant. Everyone who is left takes on more duties, and they may or may not handle those new duties, in addition to their old ones, efficiently and effectively. Studies of the natural course of change following brain injury demonstrate that partial recovery of function can and does occur (Wilson, 1998b). And there is increasing evidence that interventions, such as re-training or compensatory aids, can result in improved cognitive functioning, thereby reducing the everyday consequences of cognitive deficits and the extent to which these problems interfere with social and emotional functioning.

Following stroke the possibility of brain functions being improved through re-training opens the door to new technologies and therapies for rehabilitation of stroke survivors that have the potential to substantially reduce both amount and length of one-on-one treatment. However, any observable gains from these technological interventions need to be supported by scientific evidence of the mechanisms underlying these changes for new treatments to be widely adopted. This is where the experimental psychologist steps in.

Hypothesis testing

Every scientific investigation begins with one or more hypotheses to be tested. In fact, psychologists, as other scientists, rely on the scientific method – a systematic approach to gathering information, while adhering to certain values and standards such as:

Accuracy: gathering information in as careful and errorless a manner as possible;

161

Objectivity: obtaining, analyzing, and interpreting information in as unbiased a way as possible;

Skepticism: accepting findings as accurate only after they have been verified through repeated studies and by many different experimenters working independently of one another;

Open-mindedness: changing one's views when new evidence shows these views to be inaccurate.

All hypothesis testing is theory driven, meaning that it relies on a basic framework for explaining events or experiences. The typical sequence of events in hypothesis testing usually goes like this:

First, a theory is developed based on existing evidence. This theory helps to take existing information and organise it in a way that new predictions about behaviour can be made.

Second, these predictions – hypotheses – are then tested by further research.

Third, if the results support the theory it is strengthened and if not, the theory is modified and more testing is done.

Finally, after these rigorous procedures, the theory is either accepted as accurate or rejected as inaccurate. If it is accepted, however, it remains open to further testing and refinement as more research is done.

Errorless learning

Hypothesis: Errorless learning will be more effective for remediating post-stroke deficits in attention and executive/ motor functions than trial-and-error learning. This is the hypothesis we set out to test in a series of experiments with stroke patients with cognitive deficits. But why this hypothesis instead of its alternative that trial-and-error learning would be more effective? After all, we all know the old adage 'we learn from our mistakes'. What is the theory behind our hypothesis?

Memory for material learned without errors has been most often attributed to implicit memory. This is the kind of memory that you are not consciously aware of or would have difficulty explaining if asked to do so – like how to tie your shoes. Most people know how to do this but have difficulty explaining how. Showing is easier than telling. Baddeley and Wilson (1994) proposed that one of the major functions of explicit memory – memory you are consciously aware of – is the elimination of learning errors. This type of memory is facilitated by devoting full attention to the material to be remembered. In contrast, responses based on implicit memory depend on the strongest response given. If erroneous responses are allowed to occur they are then strengthened across repeated learning experiences.

While people with intact cognitive abilities are able to learn from their mistakes, research in the field of cognitive rehabilitation with memory impairments has demonstrated that conscious awareness during learning is important for error correction to occur. For many individuals with brain injury, this conscious awareness or explicit memory of the learning event, is diminished or simply not available. The initial response given is typically unconsciously remembered and repeated, regardless of whether it is a correct response. For example, if the stroke patient is unable to remember the name of her physiotherapist and is encouraged to guess the name, if she says the wrong name, that is the one that may be remembered and repeated. Once this error response has been established it is very difficult to

163

'unlearn.' We already knew from a number of other studies that errorless learning is particularly effective for people with memory impairments following brain injury (Wilson et al, 1994; Wilson and Evans, 1996). Given the prevalence of memory problems following stroke, we hypothesized errorless learning would be more effective in rehabilitating other types of cognitive deficits such as unilateral spatial neglect.

For errorless learning to be successful the procedures need to be 'foolproof', with learning tasks kept simple, guessing discouraged, and correct responses provided before the individual has a chance to make an error. A variety of techniques have been employed to prevent errors from being made during the learning process. For example, 'forward chaining' involves learning the first step of the task correctly before the second and subsequent steps are taught. 'Backward chaining' takes a reverse approach in which all steps of the task are completed with prompts followed by gradually withdrawing prompts, from the last step then subsequent steps, in reverse order of their occurrence in the task.

To implement errorless learning that would be 'foolproof' we decided to turn to technology to assist in our investigation. Our study employed force feedback technology. This technology is currently being used in a broad range of activities from the powered joysticks used with computer games to, for example, feel like a machine gun rapidly firing, to pilot simulation training which can mimic the feel characteristics of the steering mechanism during high speed flight. For our study, force feedback was delivered through an active joystick powered by a computer controlled electronic gearbox (more detailed description below) to implement errorless learning in our participants.

Response-guided errorless learning with elderly

Hypothesis: errorless training will result in faster and more accurate judgments in a perceptual motor task with normal elderly than trial-and-error training.

Before training any stroke patients with errorless learning using force feedback equipment, we did what is quite common in experimental psychology − first we tried our method with neurologically normal individuals. We investigated the use of response guidance for errorless learning of a perceptual motor task in a healthy elderly population without neurological problems. It provided normative data for the second study with stroke patients, using the same technique for cognitive rehabilitation.

We knew errorless learning had been shown to be more effective than trial-and-error learning on a range of tasks for people with memory impairments, but its use with normal individuals had received limited attention. Our questions were (1) whether errorless training of a perceptual motor task was more effective for improving and retaining accuracy; and (2) whether both accuracy and response speed were more resilient to the effects of increased cognitive demands.

A sample of 43 normal elderly in the United Kingdom, ranging in age from 60 to 77, completed a paper-and-pencil assessment of intelligence, memory, and attention. Each participant then received training, over two sessions, on a perceptual motor learning task − line bisection of the Judd Arrow (Judd, 1899) − which has been reliably shown to produce a misperception of the midpoint of the arrow's shaft in the direction of the arrow tail (see Figure 1). We selected this figure as representative of the perceptual error that a stroke patient with unilateral spatial neglect might experience in not attending to all aspects of what their eyes are seeing. The arrows were presented one at a time on a computer screen (see Figure 2). Participants held an active force feedback (AFF) joystick (see Figure 3) and used it to position a red cross-shaped cursor on the screen over the midpoint of the horizontal section of each arrow.

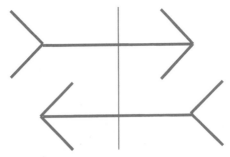

Figure 1. Judd arrow figure with true midpoint marked with vertical line.

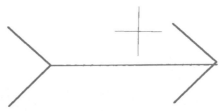

Figure 2. Computer screen with Judd arrow and cross cursor used to bisect arrow.

Participants were divided into two groups. During training, the errorless (EL) group received AFF guidance to the correct midpoint, while the errorful (EF) group received no guidance. Guidance by the AFF system involved setting a force field 'valley' around a straight line path from start point to the arrow shaft midpoint. Although the participant had to make an active movement along the direction of the valley, the valley ensured the movement path would be straight to the target and, importantly, without error. Both

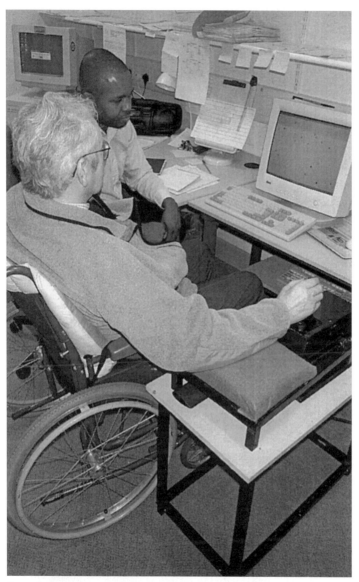

Figure 3. Patient using AFF joystick, computer and arm rest during visuospatial task.

EL and EF groups received auditory knowledge of results to let them know with a pleasant 'bell' tone if they marked the midpoint and an unpleasant 'clanging' tone if they missed. There was no AFF guidance during baseline when we were observing what their normal accuracy and response speed was before training. And there was no AFF guidance when we measured their performance following training. Training in each of the two sessions was to a criterion based on each individual's performance when bisecting plain lines on the computer using the joystick with no AFF guidance. There was a discontinue rule if accuracy did not improve. At the end of the second session both groups were given a cognitively challenging task to do concurrently with bisecting the arrows.

Results revealed that both groups improved their accuracy through training. Figure 4 for left-pointing arrows and

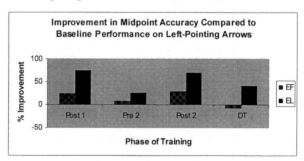

Figure 4.

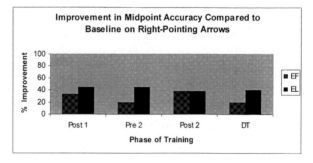

Figure 5.

Figure 5 for right-pointing arrows show accuracy for the two groups at each phase of training, compared to their initial pre-training performance. While each individual was given the same instructions on each block of trials – 'work as quickly and accurately as you can' – the EF group's response speed did not change as a result of training. The EL group was significantly faster than the EF group under the cognitive challenge without sacrificing their accuracy advantage. These results suggested that the force feedback guidance was an effective means of implementing errorless perceptual motor learning, and encouraged us to move forward with using this system with stroke patients.

Cognitive rehabilitation using response guided errorless learning with stroke patients

Hypothesis:errorless training will result in faster and more direct movements to targets in a visuospatial task for stroke patients with visual perceptual deficits.

This project was funded by the British Stroke Association. In this 18-month-long project, 19 independently living, community based male and female patients, ranging in age from 38 to 83, from the United Kingdom participated 12 months or more after their stroke. These individuals were recruited through a variety of sources, including geriatricians in local health authorities, stroke clubs (community based support groups), and the University of Birmingham, School of Psychology, patient panel of volunteers. No patient was refused entry into the study on the basis of the nature or the severity of their post-stroke deficits. And the severity of individual deficits was not equally distributed across the groups. Each of the19 patients was assigned to one of three types of training depending on the specific nature of their most prominent cognitive problem. The three types of training were visuospatial (where things are located in space), auditory-verbal memory (memory for what you hear and read), and lexical decision-making (is this group of letters that look like a word really a word?). So far we have analyzed data for the visuospatial task and the data for the other two training types is ongoing.

Twelve of the 19 patients, who showed some form of visual perceptual processing difficulty, were assigned to the visuospatial training task. The number and severity of the patients' visuospatial deficits ranged from minor visual memory problems to profound impairments across all of the paper-and pencil neuropsychological assessments, including severe unilateral spatial neglect. The training tasks, which were designed to improve visuospatial skills, involved following a trail through an array of letters of the alphabet displayed on the computer screen interspersed among star-shaped distractors. These letters were to be marked in order. There were gaps in the target letter or number strings, for example A,B,D,F,H,L,M. This required the patient to maintain in working memory (the kind of memory used when the telephone operator gives the phone number you want to ring and you have nothing to write it on) the previously marked target while locating the next one in order.

A cross-over design was used in which each individual received both EF and EL training on similar but different tasks. Half of the patients received EF training first followed by EL, and the other half received EL first followed by EF. Patients were assigned to either the EF training first (group 1) or EL training first (group 2) based on alternating the training type as each individual completed the pre-training phase during which we collected data on their 'normal' performance on the tasks on which they would later be trained. This pre-training phase involved one hour per session, one day per week, for three weeks. Originally, six patients were allocated to each group however, two patients in group 2 did not complete the second training, and two patients in group 1 had only minor visual memory problems, with no other visuospatial problems. These two 'flies in the experimental ointment' caused we, the experimenters, some problems which you will see shortly.

Following the pre-training data collection phase, each patient was trained for one hour per day, one day per week, for four weeks in one type of training. This was followed by three weeks of collecting performance information on the same tasks that the patients performed in the pre-training phase. Afterward, each person was trained for one hour per day, one day per week, for four weeks in the alternate type of training. The AFF joystick and computer used in the normal elderly study were also used in this study (see Figure 3). All patients used their unimpaired arm and hand to move the joystick.

As in the Judd Arrow experiment with the normal elderly, patients had to move the on-screen cross cursor between targets displayed on the computer screen (ignoring the distractors). They made their target selections by depressing a button on top of the joystick. During training they received both visual (a red tick mark) and auditory (pleasant 'bell' for correct and unpleasant 'clang' for incorrect) knowledge of results on each target. In the guided or EL training the AFF joystick system defined a 'force field valley' within which the joystick could be moved, which prevented movement to incorrect targets on the screen. As in the normal elderly study, while the joystick did not move the patient to the correct target, it facilitated reaching the target by generating forces that resisted movements in any direction other than a straight-line path to the correct target. In the non-guided or EF condition the joystick's force feedback was switched off allowing for unrestricted, trial-and-error movement.

In the data analysis, each patient's results were treated as a separate experiment in a single case series. This approach is one way of dealing with the problem of no stroke producing the exact same damage in any two people even though it may be in the same part of the brain in both. We analyzed the results for two aspects of the data collected: (1) response speed – the time from first button press at the beginning of each screen of targets and distracters, to final button press on the final target of that screen, and (2) perpendicular distance – the maximum deviation from the straight line path in the movement from start location to target for each target on the screen. While accuracy data were collected this information proved to be uninformative for either targets the patient might have missed or targets successfully marked. Both time and deviation from the straight line trajectory offered more useful information about improvements in visual scanning. Data were collected at three phases in the experiment: (1) pre-training, (2) at the end of the first training type, which was also prior to beginning the second training type, and (3) following the second training type. At each phase of the experiment the task changed across five combinations of targets (T) and distracters (D): 7 T–7 D, 5 T–10 D, 7 T–14 D, 13 T–20 D, and 20 T–20 D.

Figures 6 and 7 below show the response time performance of two patients who, on entry into the project, showed significant deficits in performance on all neuro-psychological tests of visual perception. Both patients showed evidence of profound impairment on visual memory and processing speed measures. On paper and pencil letter-trailmaking both patients were unable to hold onto the

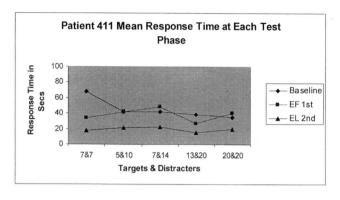

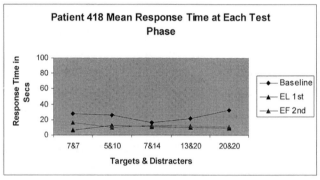

Figures 6 and 7.

concept of shifting from numbers to letters in a continuous string (1–A, 2–B, 3–C, 4–D), showing obvious confusion about the sequencing on this task. For patient 411 errorful training was completed first and for patient 418 errorless training was first in order. For both, the type of training had a significant effect on response speed in favor of the EL training. Errorless training resulted in a significant improvement in response speed that was maintained across all levels of difficulty, compared to pre-training performance. Training also produced more consistent straight line trajectories to targets across all levels of target and distracter combinations for patient 418 but had no effect on the variability of the trajectories for patient 411.

A statistical analysis was carried out comparing group 1 with group 2. This analysis was not terribly informative for several reasons. For group statistical analyses to be effective, it is necessary to have sufficient numbers in each group to show an effect, and the groups need to be as similar as possible in both size and composition. Our efforts were limited by small group size from the outset (6 in each group), unequal group sizes at completion (6 in group1 and 4 in group 2), and heterogeneity of groups (the two least impaired were in group 1 and the one most impaired was in group 2). We are currently examining two relevant aspects of unilateral spatial neglect in this study: left versus right visual field presentation of targets and line bisection. If we find that patients who had unilateral spatial neglect prior to training are now more effective and efficient at finding targets on the left side of the screen and bisecting the middle of horizontal lines following training, then we will have some evidence to support that training did improve this cognitive problem.

Statistics are not the only means of measuring improvement as a result of an experimental intervention. For some patients there are changes that simply cannot be reduced to quantifiable numbers. We call this clinical significance, in contrast to statistical significance. From a clinical standpoint, we have observable evidence that patients who did not show statistically significant improvement have experienced improvement in their daily lives. Since participating in training, one individual resumed water colour painting as a hobby, which she had been unable to do post-stroke because her visual perception and action was disorganized. Another participant, a retired engineering technician with unilateral spatial neglect, was able to reduce his response speed to targets, regardless of visual field presentation, by half. And, the patient with the most profound visual perceptual deficits, who during errorful training would have difficulty maintaining attention and was observed to go to sleep on occasion when unable to find the target, showed immediate improvement in response speed at the more complex distracter levels as a result of training. The change in their daily lives, for some patients, suggests there are as yet unmeasured gains from participation in this experimental training.

Where do we go from here?

Hypothesis: Errorless learning will be more effective for remediating post-stroke deficits in attention and executive/ motor functions than trial-and-error learning.

We started with an *hypothesis* that was theory based. We designed experiments to test this hypothesis. We were as *accurate* as possible in collecting our data. We maintained *objectivity* in obtaining, analysing, and interpreting our information. Our results fail to support or refute our hypothesis – they are equivocal. Some patients benefited more from EL than EF training; some benefited more from EF than EL training, and one patient did not benefit from either! Being both *skeptical* and *open-minded* about our research, do we now abandon our hypothesis? Where do we go from here?

As scientists, we recognize there are rarely results so clean and clear cut as to be irrefutable. Given that some patients actually benefited from the EL training, we are not ready to abandon our hypothesis. So, the next step is to modify. We might modify our hypothesis, or we might modify our method of testing the hypothesis. What will we do differently next time?

There were important limitations to this research that will be remedied in subsequent work. We can consider two ways of addressing the heterogeneity of the patients' cognitive deficits. We can either choose to focus on a more homogeneous group of patients, for example those with moderate to severe unilateral spatial neglect, eliminating other post-stroke cognitive deficits; or we can develop more individualized training tasks for a variety of types of cognitive problems. If we do the former, it could take us quite some time to find enough patients to do a group comparison but there would be a common training with each person measured against the same standard. If we develop more training tasks so we can accommodate a variety of cognitive deficits, then we would have less difficulty finding enough patients and would make a substantial investment in task design and programming those tasks – which would involve much in the way of pilot testing before large scale patient training could be carried out. We could still do a group analysis with the more heterogeneous patients, but it would be based on individual difference scores pre- and post-training.

Regardless of whether we select a singular type of cognitive problem to train or a variety, one aspect of group assignment will be very important. We will want to make certain the severity of cognitive problems in our patients is equally distributed among the experimental groups. We will also want to have experimental groups large enough such that individuals dropping out of the project – attrition – will not selectively affect one group more so than the other(s). Rather than a cross-over design, we might also want to consider bringing enough patients into the study that each patient only receives one type of training. In this case, there would be no second type of training that might be influenced by the first. Additionally, we know from studies in the investigation of brain plasticity, that it takes repeated practice for lasting changes to occur.

Next time, we will definitely want patients to receive training several days a week, rather than only one, and over many weeks – massed practice. This level of participation will take a substantial commitment on the part of each patient. The risk they take is that the training will not be beneficial. However, that is the beauty of science. Each participant enters a research project recognizing he or she may not benefit directly but do so recognizing individuals similar to themselves may benefit in the future – even if the outcome is learning that a procedure is not effective which leads to abandoning that approach. While we would not like to find ourselves in the position of having to abandon our errorless learning hypothesis, as scientists we are prepared to reject it if, after continued rigorous research procedures, we find it to be inaccurate. And, if after those same rigorous research procedures we find it to be accurate, we do not stop there. We will want to know what are the circumstances in which it works best; are there conditions under which it does not work at all, and what are they? Each answer to a question is not an end to our investigation but a beginning to the next questions that need to be addressed.

References

Baddeley A D & Wilson B A. 'When implicit memory fails: amnesia and the problem of error elimination', *Neuropsychologia*, 1993, 32, pp. 53–68.

deVeber G, Roach E S, Riela A R, Wiznitzer M. 'Stroke in children: Recognition, treatment, and future directions', *Seminars in Pediatric Neurology*, 2000, 7, pp. 309–17.

Dobkin B. 'The economic impact of stroke', *Neurology*, 1995, 45 (Suppl 1), S6-S9.

177

Jeffery D R & Good D C. 'Rehabilitation of the stroke patient', *Current Opinion in Neurology*, 1995, 8, pp. 62–8.

Kwa V H I, Limburg M, & deHaan R J. 'The role of cognitive impairment in the quality of life after ischemic stroke', *Journal of Neurology*, 1996, 243, pp. 599–604.

National Stroke Association. 'Brain attack statistics', 2001. Webpage: www.stroke.org/brain_stat.cfm.

Riddoch M J & Humphreys G W. 'The effect of cueing on unilateral neglect', *Neuropsychologia*, 1983, 21, pp. 589–99.

Riddoch M J, Humphreys G W, & Bateman A. 'Cognitive deficits following stroke', *Physiotherapy*, 1995a, 81, pp. 465–72.

Starkstein S E & Robinson R G. 'Current research in affective disorders following stroke', *Journal of Neuropsychiatry*, 1990, 2, pp. 1–14.

Stroke Association 'Stroke – Facts and Figures statistics', 2001. Webpage: www.stroke.org.uk/facts.htm.

Tatemichi T K, Desmond D W, Stern Y, Paik M, Sano M, & Bagiela E. 'Cognitive impairment after stroke: Pattern and relationship to functional abilities', *Journal of Neurology, Neurosurgery, and Psychiatry*, 1994, 57, pp. 202–7.

Wilson B A, Baddelely A D, Evans J J and Shiel A. 'Errorless learning in the rehabilitation of memory impaired people', *Neuropsychological Rehabilitation*, 1994, 4, pp. 307–26.

Wilson B A, and Evans J J. 'Error free learning in the rehabilitation of individuals with memory impairments', *Journal of Head Trauma Rehabilitation*, 1996, 11, 54–64.

Wilson B A. 'Compensating for cognitive deficits', *Paper presented at the meeting of the National Academy of Neuropsychology*, Washington, D.C., 1998a.

Wilson B A. 'Recovery of functions following nonprogressive brain injury', *Current Opinion in Neurobiology*, 1998b, 8, pp. 281–7.

Please address correspondence to: Professor Alan Wing, Behavioural Brain Sciences Centre, The University of Birmingham, Edgbaston, Birmingham B15 2TT. Tel: 0121 414 7954; fax: 0121 414 4897. Email: a.m.wing@bham.ac.uk

Some final thoughts

PUTTING A BOOK together takes quite a time. You start with an idea, get it down, think and struggle some more and it gradually changes. It gains a momentum of its own until by the time it is finished it bears little resemblance to the original outline. It is sometimes rather disconcerting for the publisher but that is the only way I can work.

Recovering from a stroke bears some similarities to creating a book. You start slowly, not knowing the final outcome. With luck and some hard work your whole attitude changes. I am glad that I wrote Part 1 nearly two years ago. I could not write it now. I have moved on and no longer think the same way. It is not only that I have learned a lot from researching the subject so that other opinions would get in the way of my original observations, but I look forward not back. I no longer think of myself as disabled, certainly not in my own home – unless I see myself reflected in someone else's eyes or attitudes.

You can tell that I have written different parts of this book at different times. But where do you stop? With recovering from a stroke; probably never. Maybe I will even walk properly one day. But with a book; that is different. I keep hearing things that I want to discuss and share, but if I do not stop soon everything will be out of date before this is even published. Things are beginning to move in stroke care, attitudes are starting to change. I hope this book will add to the momentum.

Information on the internet

There is a great deal of useful information, at all levels, to be found on the internet. Here are some useful websites from a list provided by the Stroke Association

Stroke Association
    e-mail: stroke@stroke. org.uk
    website: www.stroke.org.uk

World Health Organisation
    www.who.int/whr

Medical Monitor, aimed at both GPs and patients
    www.healthinfocus.co.uk

Different Strokes
    e-mail: different@strokes.demon.co.uk
    website: www.differentstrokes.co.uk

Royal College of Physicians
    www.rcplondon.ac.uk

British Brain and Spine Foundation
    e-mail: info@bbsf.org.uk
    website: www.bbsf.org.uk

British Aphasiology Society
    www.bas.org.uk

Disability Net, for disability news and information
    www.disabilitynet.co.uk

Disability-shop. sells disability and care products
    www.disability-shop.co.uk

AbilityNet, a charity giving free advice on computer and
web use for people with disabilities
www.abilitynet.co.uk

Website bringing disability information into the
twenty-first century
www.4dp.com

Internet stroke support group
members.aol.com/scmmlm/main.html
Newsletter:
members.aol.com/scmmlm/nl.htm

Sign on-line, Scottish Intercollegiate Guidelines a network
for information about care in Scotland
show.cee.hw.ac.uk/sign/home.html

Support Groups, information on groups for almost any
illness or condition
www.patient.co.uk

British Medical Acupuncture Society, BMAS
www.medical-acupuncture.co.uk

Disability Rights Commission
www.drc-gb.org

FOR CARERS
Developed by Action for Carers & Surrey County Council
www.carersnet.org.uk

Launched by the Department of Health
www.carers.gov.uk

Charity
www.caring-matters.org.uk

FOR NURSES
Nurse Collaborative Group
dcn.ed.ac.uk.ist3

FOR HEALTH CARE PROFESSIONALS

An information centre and forum, for the exchange of views with links to other strokesites

    www.strokeforum.com/

British Association of Stroke Physicians

    e-mail: MSD@skull.dcn.ed.ac.uk

European Stroke Conference

    www.eurostroke.org

RESEARCH

Medical Research Council

    www.mrc.ac.uk

The MRC Brain Repair Centre Cambridge

    www.brc.cam.ac.uk

Society for Research into Rehabilitation

    e-mail: ann.hughes@nottingham.ac.uk

BMJ (British Medical Journal)

    Full text of all information in editions of BMJ, available free on: www.bmj.com

Index

Note: bold type indicates a whole chapter by a named contributing author

Abel, L F 81
AbilityNet 183
Action for Carers 183
Action Research 157
activities
  functional activities training 101, 103–4
  importance of 21, 80, 81, 144–5
activities in daily living (ADL) 135–6, 145, 155, 160
acupuncture 52, 155, 183
ADL see activities in daily living
adolescent/teenage stroke patients 45, 112–13
adrenalin 38
Adult Hemiplegia (Bobath) 79
AFF (active force feedback) joystick, for response-guided learning 164–9
age
  and different needs of patients 51, 111–19, 157
  children 9, 18, 111–16, 120–6, 158
  elderly/older 8, 24, 29, 62, 106, 118–19, 129–30, 134–52
  teenage/adolescent patients 45, 112–13
  younger (than elderly) patients 9, 51, 58–9, 62, 106–7, 116–17, 127–33, 155, 156
  as risk factor 158–9
aids 28, 70, 114, 131
  walking aids 37, 57–9, 72–8, 117, 145
alternative therapy 51–3
ambidexterity 40
America, depression treatment 138
anaemia 120, 121, 122, 123, 126, 158
Andrew-Withey 138
ankle 71, 73
anticoagulation/anticoagulants 124, 126
anxiety and worry 23, 37, 42, 112, 132, 135, 136
Aphasia Handbook (Connect) 156
aphasia (loss of speech) 17, 49, 84–96, 132, 136, 140, 146, 147, 156, 159
  incidence and prevalence 85, 93
  services for people with 86–8
  see also speech and language therapy; speech problems
aphasiology 63, 88, 94, 96, 182
apoplexy (stroke) 134
appetite, assessing 138
Arie, T 148

arm, function 18, 39, 44, 69, 70, 73, 75, 76, 117
aromatherapy 52
art therapy 47–8
arteriogram 122
artery, blocked 121, 122–3
arthritis 135
articulation problems (in speech) 85, 90
Asberg, M 138
aspiration pneumonia 87
aspirin, low-dose 124, 126
attention problems 97–8, 99, 117, 159, 160
attitude
  of doctors 35–6, 64, 105–8
  of friends and family 32, 36–7, 149
  of patient 15, 149
  of therapist 35, 61
  to walking aids 37
auditory-verbal memory 170
Australia
  treatment in 137, 138, 140
  University of Western Australia 58–9
Avemark, C et al 140
awareness, difficulties with 99, 142

B vitamins 123, 126
'baby boom generation' 158–9
backward chaining 164
balance 36, 50, 75, 144–5, 155
basketball 50
Bateman, A 160
bath seat 28
bed
  positioning arm in 70
  stretching to reach objects oneself 25
  turning over in 27
behavioural problems 18
Beijing 50, 52
benefits and rights information 128, 131
bereavement, comparision with stroke 36
Bernspang, B 136, 141
Birmingham University research 156, 157, 158–79
bleeding into brain (cerebral haemorrhage) 121, 123, 124
blood
  circulation/supply/flow, reduced 122, 124, 136
  clotting 121, 122

sticky 121, 122, 124, 126
tests 124
transfusion 123
vessel narrowing and obstruction 121,
    122, 123, 126
Bobath Concept 63–4, 79–83
body, neglected areas of 69–71
bones, broken 32, 36, 37
boredom 46
Botulinum toxin 70, 81, 125
Boyd, R V 149
brain
    bleeding into (cerebral haemorrhage) 121,
        123, 124
    communication processing parts 90
    damage 22, 72, 122, 123
    encephalitis (inflammation of the brain) 85
    lesion, site of 140
    reduced blood flow 122, 124, 136
    reduced oxygen 121, 122, 123
    retraining (neural plasticity) 22, 80, 160–1
    scanning 121–2
    structural abnormality 122
    surgery 123
    tumour 120
brain attack (stroke) 22
Brannagan, Anne 64, **97–104**
British Aphasiology Society 63, 88, 96, 182
British Association of Stroke Physicians 184
British Brain and Spine Foundation 182
British Medical Acupuncture Society 183
British Medical Journal (BMJ) 184
British Society of Rehabilitation Medicine
    107, 108
Bryan, Dr Karen 156
Burnard, S 148, 149
Burridge, Jane 57, **72–8**
Burvill, P et al 140
bypass surgery 124

calf tone, increase in 73
cancer 127
cancer patients 140
capital letters, writing 14
cardiac (heart) disease 120, 121, 126, 127,
    158
careers, effect of stroke on 106
carers
    help for 102, 103, 104, 131, 146–7, 183
    role of 30–1, 46, 68, 69, 94, 118, 119
    'carry-over' effect 57–8, 74, 75
Cast, Jane 37, 43, 59–61, **65–71**
Catie Learns to Draw (Roberts) 47–8
causes of childhood stroke 120–1
cerebral haemorrhage (bleeding into brain)
    121, 123, 124
cerebral palsy 72

chair, posture and movement 29, 70–1
charities
    individual grants from 131
    research funding 155–7
cheerfulness 24, 37–8
cheque signing 16
Chest Heart & Stroke Scotland, The 156
chickenpox 121, 122, 126
childhood stroke 9, 18, 111–16, 120–6,
    155, 158
choice indicator board/chart 17, 26
choking 27
cholesterol, high 122, 126
church, motivation to go to 32
Clinical Rehabilitation journal 107
clock test, drawing the 141
clumsiness 31
CNS (central nervous system) 63–4, 80
co-ordination 50
cognition, definition 97
cognitive neuro-psychological theory 89, 9
cognitive problems 97–104, 146, 147, 159–
Cognitive Rehabilitation Therapy 64, 100–
    117, 156
    response-guided learning 158–79
cold, extreme 34
College of Health 118
communication
    by gesture 92
    with choice indicator board/chart 17, 26
    problems with 17, 21, 26, 43, 49, 85,
        92–3, 132, 146
community (out-patient) physiotherapy
    34–5, 65–71, 149
complications, secondary 69
comprehension, (understanding) reading an
    listening 85, 91, 92, 98, 159
compromise, during rehabilitation 31, 33
computer
    for learning and entertainment 50, 62
    writing with 40
computer game technology 164
computer games for older people 50
computer-assisted tomography (CT) scannin
    121, 122
computer-based exercises 100, 102
computer-based research experiment 156,
    158–79
concentration 97, 132, 140
confidence 16, 26, 30, 47, 75, 100
Connect 49, 87, 93, 156
constipation 146
contractures 70
conversation partners 93, 94
conversations, difficulty with 91, 98
cooking 32, 40, 103
coping ability 135

correspondence, managing 91
cost, reduced, by home rehabilitation 149
costs of education and lost productivity 158
counselling 23, 93, 128, 129, 146
courtesy, need for 32
cramp, writer's (dystonia) 19
cramps 27
crying, uncontrollable 132
CT (computer-assisted tomography) scanning 121, 122
Curtin University, Australia 59

D-T (delighted-terrible) face scale 137–40
daily life, speech problems and 89, 91
daily living, activities in (ADL) 135–6, 145, 155, 160
daily living skills 31, 40–1, 62
Daily Telegraph, The 20
Damiano, D L 81
darts 50
day, planning your 33–4
day care 148
day centres 46, 130
de Haan, R J 160
de Veber, G, et al 158
Dean, 144
decisions, making 32
Defence Services Rehabilitation Centre, Headley Court 64
Delighted-Terrible (D-T) face scale 137–40
Denmark, muscle stimulator from 75–6
dental checkups 33, 39
Department of Health 118, 183
dependence on others 16, 25, 31
depression
    avoiding 15, 16, 37, 46, 67, 148
    causes of 22–3, 53, 134, 136–40, 160
    masked 138–40
determination 32–3
diary of progress, keeping 27
diet, balanced 124, 126
Different Strokes 9, 51, 64, 115, 116–17, 131
    details 127–9, 133, 156, 182
dignity 25, 47
disability, stigma of 129
Disability Net 182
Disability Rights Commission 183
Disability-shop 182
distance judgement, impaired 142
distractions, ignoring background 97
district nurses 35
divorce 140
dizzy, feeling 44
Dobkin, B 159
doctors
    GPs 35–6
    hospital 105–7, 108

dorsiflexion (foot lift) 73, 75
drawing 141
    as communication 49
    one-sided 47, 143, 160
dressing yourself 23, 25, 44, 125
    one-sided 143
drinking, problems with 26–7, 147
driving 41, 59
drop foot 42, 72, 73–5
drugs 81, 125
    anti-depressive 140
drunk, stroke symptom ascribed to being 129
dysarthria (functional speech problem) 85
dysphagia (swallowing problem) 26–7, 85, 86–7
dysphonia (voice impairment) 85
dyspraxia (disturbance of voluntary movement) 27, 85
dystonia (writer's cramp) 19, 27

Eastern Motor Group 13
eating
    one-sided 160
    problems with 26–7, 44, 147
Ebrahim, S et al 135
ECG (electrocardiogram) 122
echocardiogram (ECHO) 122
education, effect on 9, 111, 125, 129, 158
education of patients, about rehabilitation 100, 101–2, 128
Ehrsson, H H et al 64
elderly/older people
    needs of 8, 24, 29, 62, 106, 118–19, 129–30, 134–52
    posture 144
    response-guided learning with 165–9
electric gadgets 39
electrical stimulation of nerves/muscles see functional electrical stimulation (FES)
electrocardiogram (ECG) 122
electrodes 73
emotions/feelings of patients, respect for 8, 91, 93, 97, 119, 129, 132, 135
employment, returning to 32, 117, 128, 129, 156
encephalitis (inflammation of the brain) 85
encouragement 19, 21, 22, 33, 37, 53, 67, 68, 147
energy, conserving 33–4, 40
Ericsson, Professor Kjerstin 119, **134–52**
errorless learning, explanation 162–4
ethnography 94
European Stroke Conference 184
Evans, J J 164
Evans, R L, et al 149
evening, best or worst time of day 34
eversion (foot twisting outwards) 75

everyday life
  activities in daily living (ADL) 135–6,
    145, 155, 160
  skills 31, 40–1, 62
  speech problems and 89, 91
executive functions 99, 117
exercise 16, 41, 52, 70, 76
  for children 124, 126
  classes 127, 130
  computer-based 100, 102
  self-prescribed (as therapy) 41, 44–5
  swimming 41, 44, 50, 127
  when (part of day) to do 34
Exeter University research 155
explanation of stroke to patients 22, 23, 42,
  69, 71
extremes of hot and cold 34
eye checkups 33
eye problems 98

Factor V Leiden 122, 124, 126
falling over and tripping 30, 31, 32, 36, 72,
  73, 75, 144
family/relatives
  attitude of 32, 36–7, 149
  help for 22, 28, 114, 146–7
  help from 33, 94, 120, 145, 149
fatigue 112, 149
fats (lipids), high levels of 122, 124, 126
fear 27, 42, 67, 132
feelings/emotions of patients, respect for 8,
  91, 93, 97, 119, 129, 132, 135
FES see functional electrical stimulation
fibula 73
fingers 22
Flament, D et al 64
flu 41
folic acid 123, 126
food
  balanced diet 124, 126
  choice of 124, 126
  cooking 32, 40, 103
  eating problems 26–7, 44, 147
  going too long without 41
  meals delivered to home 28
  swallowing 26
foot
  exercise for 52
  functional electrical stimulation for 57–9,
    72–8, 117
  twisting outwards (eversion) 75
foot drop see drop foot
foot lift (dorsiflexion) 73, 75
footwear, appropriate 37, 71
force feedback technology 164
force field valley 166, 171
force output 81

form filling 16
Forster, A 149
forward chaining 164
friends and family, attitude of 32, 36–7
fruit, eating 124, 126
frustration 18, 30, 31, 38, 43
functional activities training 101, 103–4
functional electrical stimulation (FES) 58–9
  70, 72–8, 81

gadgets 39, 131
gait 70, 71, 73, 75, 144
gait analysis 58–9, 61
gardening 41
genetic predisposition to stroke 121, 123,
  124, 158
genetic testing 122
geometrical figures, copying 141
geriatric care see elderly/older people
gesture, use for communication 92
Gladman, J R F, et al 149
Glasgow research 117, 156
Glossop, E S 149
gluteus maximus muscle 75
goals, difficulty setting appropriate 99
goals for recovery 35–6, 63–4, 66, 67, 80, 13
Good, D C 160
GPs (general practitioners) 35–6
grandchildren, motivation to visit 32
grants from charities, for individuals 131
gratitude, need for 32
gripping, with hand 39, 73

hamburgers 124
Hamer, Pete 59
hamstrings 75
hand
  electrical stimulation exercise for 73, 76
  gripping 39, 73
  one-handedness 62, 69, 113
  use of preferred and non-preferred 13,
    14–15, 18, 25, 39–40
handling techniques 70, 79, 80
handwriting 13–19, 40, 48, 49, 113
Harding, Deborah 63, **84–96**
head injuries/trauma 72, 85, 101, 126
Headway 87
health, self-perceived 135, 136
health professionals 119, 131, 184
heart, clots in 121, 122
heart (cardiac) disease 120, 121, 127, 158
heat, extreme 34
help
  accepting 25, 30, 60
  helping yourself 21, 23, 25–6, 30, 42, 6(
  see also carers; family/relatives; informatior
    resources

helpline for parents, lack of 115
hemiparesis (weakness/paralysis on one side) 121, 159
HFD (human figure drawing) 141
Hier, D B, et al 143
hip 71, 72
hip extension 75
Hippocrates 134
Holland, muscle stimulator from 75
Holmén, K et al 137, 138
home
    preparing for going 28–9
    rehabilitation at 28–9, 30–2, 67–8, 118, 119, 147–8
    trial day or night at 28
homocysteine 122, 123, 126
hope 44, 45–6, 53, 68
'hosepipe theory' 90
Hospital Anxiety and Depression Index 74
hospital doctors 105–7, 108
hospital treatment
    access to 20
    author's experience of 20–9
    discharge from 28–9, 118, 129
    ength of stay 28, 148
    speech and language therapy 87
housebound, computers and the 50
household tasks (daily living skills) 31, 40–1, 62
housing 129
human figure drawing (HFD) 141
humerus 76
Humphreys, G W 160
hunger, effect on memory and movement 41
hydrotherapy 50
    see also swimming
hypercholesterolaemia (high cholesterol) 122, 126
hypertonia (increased muscle tension, tone) 80
hypothesis testing 161–2
hypoxia (deficiency of oxygen) 121, 122, 123

immune-deficiency 126
implanted drop foot stimulator/systems 75, 76–7
incontinence 132, 147
independent living 118, 128, 130, 134, 144
indignity 25, 47
individual needs 8, 33, 62, 67, 69, 116, 130
infection 34, 85, 121, 122
inferred meaning, understanding 85
information
    available on the internet 43, 182–4
    importance of 42, 43, 67, 115, 128, 130, 131, 148
information processing 98, 99, 117
injuries 72, 85, 101, 121, 126

Institute of Child Health 115
integrated therapy 49, 53
intellect, insults to 46–7
intensive therapy, age and 118
intention, body-worn sensors to detect 76
internet, information on 43, 182–4
intervention, early 15, 24, 124
intestinal problems (constipation) 146
involuntary movement 27, 85
iron deficiency 121
Irwin, P 43
ischaemic stroke/transient ischaemic attack (mini-stroke) 85, 121
isolation 36, 51, 115, 133, 135

Jackson, J H 142
Jadback, G 136
James, Dr M 155
Jeffery, D R 160
joints 69, 70, 81
    see also ankle; hip; knee; shoulder; wrist
Joseph Rowntree Foundation 156
joysticks for response-guided learning 164–9
Judd Arrow 165–6

Karolinska Institute, Sweden 119
Kavanagh, T 149
Keele University research 157
keyboard, using computer 62
Kirkham, Dr Fenella 115–16, **120–6**
knee 71, 75
Kwa, V H I 160

Lance, J W 79
Langton Hewer, R 149
language processing 89, 90
language therapy see speech and language therapy; speech problems
laughing 23
laughter, uncontrollable 132
learning, response-guided 158–79
left hand 14–15, 18, 39
left hemisphere stroke 84, 136, 142, 159
left side of body 159–60
leg
    clotting in veins 122
    positioning of 71
    splints 37, 53
    swinging 73
    see also walking aids
leisure activities 41, 46, 135
leisure centres 130
lethargy 23
leukemia 158
lexical decision-making 170
Liberson, W T 72, 73
lifestyle changes 30, 124

Light, K E 81
limbs 24, 27
　see also arm; leg
Limburg, M 160
limp 124
Lincoln, N 149
lipids (fats), high levels of 122, 124, 126
liquids, swallowing 26–7
literature on strokes 43
living alone 29, 36, 62, 118
Lloyd, David 59
Lockwood, Richard 49
loneliness 36, 50, 51, 146
long-term care 129
lumbar puncture 122

McCrum, Robert 27
McLellan, Professor D L 64, **105–8**, 116, 155
Malia, Kit 64, **97–104**, 117
marriage, changing roles after stroke 30–1
masked depression 138–40
massage 52
Mayston, Dr Margaret 63, **79–83**
meals, delivered to home 28
Medical Monitor 182
Medical Research Council 156, 184
Medical Research Council Brain Repair Centre
　Cambridge 184
medication 23, 33, 38, 81
　advice on, and after-effects of 147
memory 99, 101, 103, 117, 132, 140, 159
　hunger and 41
　implicit and explicit 163–4
　over-tiredness and 33, 41, 112
meningitis 122, 126
Mesulam, M M 142
migraine 129
Miller, G J T 81
Milton, A, et al 148
'mind over matter' 114
mini-stroke (transient ischaemic
　attack/ischaemic stroke) 85, 121
mobility 144–5
Montgomery, S A 138
mood, assessing 136–40
morning, best or worst part of day 34
motivation 15, 21–2, 32–3, 46, 63, 145,
　146, 149
mouth, stiff lopsided 52
movement
　abrupt 27
　analysis of 81
　hunger and 41
　involuntary 27, 85
　normal sequence 159
　over-tiredness and 33, 41
　range of 70, 76

stretching 25, 27, 70, 73
　see also Bobath Concept; walking
Moyamoya (blood flow around blockage)
　123–4
MRI (Magnetic Resonance Imaging) scan
　121–2
MS (multiple schlerosis) 72
Mulley, G 148
Murray, V 138
muscles
　contraction 27
　Functional Electrical Stimulation (FES)
　　58–9, 70,72–8, 81
　overactivity 79
　stiffness (spasticity) 70, 72, 73, 74, 76,
　　79, 80
　strengthening 48, 81
　tone, increased (hypertonia) 80
　weakness (paresis) 69, 121, 140, 159
music therapy 48
My Year Off (McCrum) 27

National Academy of Neuro-psychology
　(USA) 104
National Childhood Stroke Study (Williams) 111, 1
National Clinical Guidelines on Stroke (Royal Colleg
　of Physicians) 75
National Lottery funding 156
National Service Framework (NSF) for Olde
　People 61, 118
National Stroke Association (USA) 158
'Needs of Younger Stroke Survivors and the
　Families' 156
neglect (dysfunction) 47, 48, 119, 142–3,
　160, 164, 170, 174
nerve, common peroneal 73, 75–6
nerve impulses, electrical stimulation
　replacing see functional electrical stimulatic
nervous system, central (CNS) 63–4, 80
network for parents, lack of 115
neural plasticity (retraining brain) 22, 80,
　160–1
neuro-physiotherapy 24, 34, 35, 59–61
neurological neglects (dysfunction) 47, 48,
　119, 142–3, 160, 164, 170, 174
newsletters for stroke patients 128
NHP (Nottingham Health Profile) 135–6
NHS
　benefits of wards 25
　provision of leaflets 131
　rehabilitation 106
　speech therapists 86
　underfunding 35
　use of ODFS 74
Nottingham Health Profile (NHP) 135–6
NSF (National Service Framework for Older
　People) 61, 118

Nudo, R 80
numbers, reversal of 40
Nurse Collaborative Group 184
nurses, help from 24, 25, 35
nursing homes 129, 140

occupational therapy (OT) 48, 50, 61–2,
    124–5
    pre-release home visit 28
occupations, finding new 46–50
ODFS see Odstock Dropped Foot Stimulator
Odstock 2 Channel Stimulator 75
Odstock Dropped Foot Stimulator (ODFS)
    57–9, 72–8, 117
oedema, ankle 73
official correspondence, misunderstanding of
    91
O'Kelly, Donal 116–17, **127–33**
older/elderly people
    needs of 8, 24, 29, 62, 106, 118–19,
        129–30, 134–52
    posture 144
    response-guided learning with 165–9
one-handed, managing 62, 69, 113
one-sided/unilateral neglect (dysfunction)
    47, 48, 119, 142–3, 160, 164, 170, 174
optician, checkups at 33
orthopaedic wards 24
orthotist, help from 71
OT see occupational therapy
'out of the blue' occurrence of stroke 120,
    121, 124
out-patient (community) physiotherapy
    34–5, 65–71, 149
outside the house, going 32–3, 145
over-tired, getting 33, 41, 112
Overstall, P W 144
oxygen supply, reduced (hypoxia) 121, 122,
    123

paediatrics, Bobath and 79
pain 27, 43, 69, 70, 76, 135
pain clinics 43
painting 46–7, 48
panic 31, 112
paralympics 49–50
paralysis 121, 132, 159
parents of child stroke patients 114, 115
paresis (muscle weakness) 69, 121, 140, 159
partners, coping by 30–1, 118
Partridge, C 149
patients, explanation of stroke to 22, 23, 42,
    69, 71
patient's role in recovery see help
PCI (Physiological Cost Index) 74, 75
pen, using a 14
    see also handwriting

Penhale, B 43
perception 119, 140–2, 147, 159
peroneal nerve 73, 75, 76
personal correspondence, inability to manage
    91
phonology (word sounds) 90
physical management plan for daily life 43,
    65–71
Physiological Cost Index (PCI) 74, 75
physiotherapy 24, 53, 65–71, 124, 145
    neuro-physiotherapy 24, 34, 35, 59–61
    out-patient (community) 34–5, 65–71,
        149
pillows, placing of 24
pilot simulation training 164
planning, difficulties with 99
plateau, reaching and going beyond a 35, 38,
    41, 42, 45, 65
platelets, increased 126
playground, help for child patients in 125
pneumonia, aspiration 87
polyclinic treatment 148
positioning aids 70
posture 29, 70–1, 144
predisposition to stroke 121, 123, 124, 158
privacy 25
private medical care 25, 49, 53
process training 100, 102–3
productivity, lost 158
progress
    measures of 39
    planning in advance 42–3
    record-keeping of 27–8
    time limit/plateau on 35, 38, 41, 42, 45,
        65
Prothrombin....20210 126
psychiatric problems 8
psychological impact of stroke 129, 131
psychological needs/problems 8, 9, 53
psychosocial impact of aphasia 93
public wards 25

quadriceps spasticity 74
quality of life 74, 86–7, 119, 134–6, 148, 160

radio, enjoyment of 91
reaching, balance while 144
reaching objects yourself 25
reading and listening comprehension
    problems 85, 91, 92, 98, 159
recipes, inability to follow 91
recognising objects 141
record-keeping of progress 27–8
recovery
    goals for 35–6, 63–4, 66, 67, 80, 130
        time limit/plateau 35, 38, 41, 42, 45, 65
    monitoring 35–6, 45–6, 130

recreation 49
Recreation and Disability in Australia (Lockwood) 49
referral system, open 35, 87
reflex activity 73, 79, 81
reflexology 52
regression, temporary 34
rehabilitation
    Cognitive Rehabilitation Therapy 64,
        100–4, 117, 156
        response-guided learning 158–79
    delayed 15, 24
    home 28–9, 30–2, 67–8, 118, 119, 147–8
    involvement of patients in planning and
        development
    see also therapy; treatment
rehabilitation medicine 106–8
relationship, changing roles after stroke 30–1
relationships and sex, advice on 131
relatives/family
    attitude of 32, 36–7, 149
    help for 22, 28, 114, 146–7
    help from 33, 94, 120, 145, 149
relaxation techniques 52
Research into Ageing 157
research projects 155–7
resources (references) for cognitive
    rehabilitation 101–4
response-guided learning experiment 156,
    158–79
    conclusions 175–7
rest 23, 44
    see also sleep
Riddoch, M J 160
right hand 14–15, 18
right hemisphere stroke 85, 159–60
right side of body 159
rights and benefits information 128, 131
risk, calculated, during recovery 37
risk factors 140, 158
    for children 121, 123, 126, 158
Roberts, Barbara 47–8
Robinson, R G 160
roles at home, changing 30–1
rolling, to help trunk 71
Rowntree (Joseph) Foundation 156
Royal College of Physicians 61, 75, 182
Royal College of Speech and Language
    Therapists 63, 87
Rudd, Dr A 43

safety 28, 32–3, 37
Salisbury District Hospital 57, 72, 77, 117
salt-laden foods 124, 126
Sassoon, Rosemary
    experience of hospital treatment 20–9
    recovery and suggestions 39–53
sausages 124

scanning of brain 121–2
school, child stroke patients and 9, 111, 12
    129, 158
school leavers, disabled 106
Scotland, treatment in 117
Scottish Intercollegiate Guidelines 183
Secombe, Sir Harry 48
self-awareness 100
self-confidence 16, 26, 30, 47, 75, 100
self-esteem 51, 100
self-help 21, 23, 25–6, 30, 42, 60
self-help groups 50–1
self-monitoring of speech and other problem
    91, 99
semantics 90
sensation, loss of 70
sensors, body-worn, to detect intention 76
sex life, effect on 135
sex and relationships, advice on 131
Shepherd 144
shoe splint 73
shoes, appropriate 37, 71
shopping 40, 62, 103
shoulder dislocation (subluxation) 70, 76
shower, hot 27
shower seat 61
siblings, effect of stroke on 114
sick, feeling 44
sickle cell (anaemia) disease 120, 121, 122
    123, 126, 158
sighing 23
Sign on-line 183
signature, ability to write 16, 62
sitting balance 144–5
sitting posture 70–1
skills for daily living 31, 40–1, 62
skills (process) training for cognitive
    difficulties 100
skin probe 122
sleep
    disturbed, due to worry 112, 135
    need for 23, 44
    patterns of, assessing 138
    study, test for child stroke patients 122
    turning over during 27
Smith, D S 149
snoring 122
social impact of stroke 129, 135, 136
social services, information on 131
social support 146
Society for Cognitive Rehabilitation, USA 64
    104
Society for Research into Rehabilitation 107
    184
South and West Development and Evaluatio
    Committee 74
South West Kent Primary Care Trust 61

Southampton General Hospital research 64, 115
spasms (involuntary movement)27 85
spasticity (muscle stiffness) 70, 72, 73, 74, 76, 79, 80
spatial perception 160
spatial unilateral neglect (dysfunction) 47, 48, 119, 142–3, 160, 164, 170, 174
Speakability 87
Speaking Out About Stroke Services (Stroke Association) 8, 118
special educational needs 125
SPECT (single photon emission computed tomography) scan 122
speech and language therapy 13–14, 43, 53, 63, 84–96, 125, 146
speech problems
    over-tiredness and 33
    slower speech 40
speech loss (aphasia) 17, 23, 49, 84–96, 132, 136, 140, 146, 147, 156, 159
    WHO classifications of 89, 91
spelling problems 89, 91
spinal cord injuries 72
spinal fluid, abnormal 122
spirit 47
splint 37, 70, 73, 74, 81
sport 49, 103
sports therapy 50
stairs and steps, managing 29, 32, 112, 145
stance, asymmetric 144
standing 24, 145
Starkstein, S E 160
started, getting, difficulties with 99
statement of educational needs 125
statistics on strokes 85, 93, 127, 158, 159
sticks, using 37, 71
stiffness
    in joints 70
    in muscles (spasticity) 70, 72, 73, 74, 76, 79, 80
stomach problems 146
Stone, M 149
straightening limbs 24, 27
strategy training 100
strength, assessing 138
stretch reflex 73, 79
stretching 25, 27, 70, 73
stroke, WHO definition 134
Stroke Association 8, 26, 87, 118, 157, 158, 169
    details 43, 51, 155–6, 182
Stroke At Our Fingertips (Rudd, Irwin, Penhale) 43
Stroke Care – A Matter of Chance (Stroke Association) 20, 118
stroke clubs (community-based support groups) 50–1

stroke support group, internet 183
Study to Evaluate the Met and Unmet Needs of Young Stroke Survivors (McLellan, et al) 116, 155
support groups 115, 183
Surrey County Council 183
Surrey University research 156
survival rates 158, 159
swallowing problem (dysphagia) 26–7, 85, 86–7
Sweden, research and treatment in 136, 138–9
Swift, Dr Peter 115
swimming, exercises while 41, 44, 50, 127
symbolism 93
symptoms of stroke
    invisible 131–3, 136
    misunderstanding of 129

Talking about Aphasia (Connect) 156
Tatemichi, T K, et al 159
Taylor, Paul 57, **72–8**
tea making 62
tears, uncontrollable 132
teenage/adolescent stroke patients 45, 112–13
teeth, caring for 33, 39
telephone, using 91
television
    enjoyment of 91
    watching 98, 103
temperament, assessing 138
tests for childhood stroke 121–2
Tham, K 142
therapy
    availability of out-patient 34–5
    delayed 15, 24
    integrated 49, 53
    self-prescribed exercises as 41, 44–5
    tiring and awkward tasks as useful 23, 25, 44–5
    see also under different types: physiotherapy; speech therapy, etc; treatment
There is Life after Stroke (Daily Telegraph) 20
thinking 132, 159
    better organised, deeper 40
    making sense of thoughts 97
    slowly and unclearly 98
tibialis anterior 73
time signposts (for recovery/plateau) 35, 38, 41, 42, 45, 65
times of the day, energy levels at different 33–4
tin-opener, electric 39
tiredness 23, 38
    getting over-tired 33, 41, 112
    tiring and awkward tasks as useful 23, 25, 44–5

toes, exercise for 52
tone 70, 73, 79
tonic stretch reflex activity 73, 79, 81
tonsillitis 121, 122, 126
toothbrush, electric 39
training
    functional activities 101, 103–4
    process (skills) 100
    strategy 101
    for work 128
transient ischaemic attack (mini-stroke) 85,
    121
trauma 121
treatment
    availability 43, 52, 86, 117
        at home 28, 67–8
        in hospital 20–9, 28, 48, 66, 67, 68, 88
        as out-patient (community) 34–5,
            65–71, 149
    see also therapy and its individual types
trial-and-error learning 162–3
triceps muscle 75
tripod, using 71
tripping and falling over 30, 31, 32, 36, 72,
    73, 75, 144
trunk, care of 70–1
typefaces, helpful 40

understanding, reading and listening 85, 91,
    92, 98, 159
unilateral neglect 47, 48, 119, 142–3, 160,
    164, 170, 174
uselessness, feeling of 46

vegetables, eating 124, 126
veins, clotting in leg 122
video recording of progress 27–8
Viitanen, M, et al 135
vision
    checkups 33
    poor, blurred or double 98, 132, 142
visitors 23, 36, 38
visual processing 98, 117
visuospatial training 170
vitamin intake 123
voice problems 85
    see also speech problems
voluntary range of movement 76

Wade, D T 149
walking
    aids for 37, 57–9, 72–8, 117, 145

learning to 66, 69, 124, 145
    speed 57, 59, 73, 74, 75
washing, hanging out the 44
weakness
    in joints 69
    in muscles 69, 121, 140, 159
websites, list of useful 182–4
weekend therapy, lack of 28
weight bearing 71, 75, 144
weight gain 135
welfare officers 146
wellbeing, assessing 137–40
West Kent Neuro-rehabilitation Unit 63
wheelchairs 25–6, 28, 36, 37, 50, 66, 71
whistling 52
White, Dr A R 155
WHO (World Health Organisation) 134,
    182
        classifications of speech problems 89, 9
William Harvey Hospital, Ashford 157
Williams, Dr A N 111, 155
Wilson, B A 160, 161, 164
Wing, Professor Alan 13, 156, 179
    et al **158–79**
Wittenstein Aktiv Technologies Ltd 158
words
    finding the right 91, 98
    meanings (semantics) 90
    sounds (phonology) 90
    understanding single 92
work, returning to 32, 117, 128, 129, 156
'Work after Stroke' 117, 156
worksheets, making activities a therapy
    103–4
World Health Organisation (WHO) 134, 18
    classifications of speech problems 89, 91
worry and anxiety 23, 37, 42, 112, 132,
    135, 136
wrist 22
writer's cramp (dystonia) 19, 27
writing 13–19, 40, 48, 49, 113
    by computer 40
    slowly 91

yawning 23
Young, J B 149
younger (than elderly) patients
    problems of 9, 51, 106–7, 116–17,
        127–33, 155, 156
        see also childhood stroke; Different
            Strokes; teenage/adolescent patients